Contents

KW-935-472

The National Collaborating Centre

for Chronic Conditions

Funded to produce guidelines for the NHS by NICE

ATRIAL FIBRILLATION

National clinical guideline for management in primary and secondary care

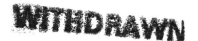

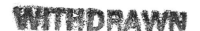

Published by

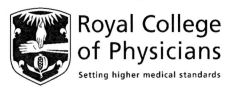

Royal College
of Physicians
Setting higher medical standards

Acknowledgements

The Guideline Development Group would like to thank the following people for their valuable input during the development of this guideline:

Mr Steven Barnes, Mrs Susan Clifford, Mr Rob Grant, Dr Bernard Higgins, Ms Jane Ingham, Ms Ester Klaeijsen, Dr Ian Lockhart, Ms Louise Martin, Ms Jill Parnham.

Mission statement

The Royal College of Physicians plays a leading role in the delivery of high quality patient care by setting standards of medical practice and promoting clinical excellence. We provide physicians in the United Kingdom and overseas with education, training and support throughout their careers. As an independent body representing over 20,000 Fellows and Members worldwide, we advise and work with government, the public, patients and other professions to improve health and healthcare.

The National Collaborating Centre for Chronic Conditions

The National Collaborating Centre for Chronic Conditions (NCC-CC) is a collaborative, multi-professional centre undertaking commissions to develop clinical guidance for the NHS in England and Wales. The NCC-CC was established in 2001. It is an independent body, housed within Clinical Standards Department at the Royal College of Physicians of London. The NCC-CC is funded by the National Institute for Health and Clinical Excellence (NICE) to undertake commissions for national clinical guidelines on an annual rolling programme.

Citation for this document

National Collaborating Centre for Chronic Conditions. *Atrial fibrillation: national clinical guideline for management in primary and secondary care.* London: Royal College of Physicians, 2006.

Copyright

ISBN 1 86016 282 7

ROYAL COLLEGE OF PHYSICIANS
11 St Andrews Place, London NW1 4LE
www.rcplondon.ac.uk

Registered charity No 210508

Typeset by Dan-Set Graphics, Telford, Shropshire

Printed in Great Britain by The Lavenham Press Ltd, Sudbury, Suffolk

APPENDICES

REFERENCES

Members of the Guideline Development Group

Dr Michael Rudolf, NCC-CC (*Chair*)
Consultant Respiratory Physician, Ealing Hospital NHS Trust

Professor Gregory Lip, NCC-CC (*Clinical Advisor*)
Professor of Cardiovascular Medicine, University Department of Medicine, City Hospital, Birmingham

Mrs Lina Bakhshi, NCC-CC
Information Scientist, Royal College of Physicians of London

Professor John Camm, British Cardiac Society
Consultant Cardiologist, St. George's Hospital Medical School, London

Dr Mark Davis, Primary Care Cardiovascular Society
General Practitioner, Moorfield House Surgery, Leeds

Mr Richard Deacon, Royal College of Nursing
Senior Charge Nurse, Leeds Teaching Hospitals NHS Trust

Dr Richard Dewar, Royal College of Physicians of London
Consultant Physician in General & Elderly Care Medicine, Pontypridd and Rhondda NHS Trust

Dr Martin Fotherby, British Geriatrics Society
Senior Lecturer in Age and Stroke Medicine, University of Leicester

Dr Jane Fisher, NCC-CC
Project Manager, Royal College of Physicians of London

Mrs Bernadette Ford, NCC-CC
Information Scientist, Royal College of Physicians of London

Dr Michael Hughes, NCC-CC
Research Fellow/Project Manager, Royal College of Physicians of London

Professor Lalit Kalra, King's College London, invited as an expert in stroke medicine to attend GDG meetings 3, 4, 11 and 14
Consultant Stroke Physician, King's College Hospital NHS Trust, London

Mr Simon Kendall, Society of Cardiothoracic Surgeons, invited as an expert in cardiothoracic surgery to attend GDG meetings 4 and 7
Consultant Cardiothoracic Surgeon, James Cook University Hospital, Middlesbrough

Dr Clifford Mann, British Association for Emergency Medicine
Consultant in Accident and Emergency Medicine, Taunton and Somerset NHS Trust

Dr Duncan McRobbie, Royal Pharmaceutical Society
Principal Clinical Pharmacist, Guy's and St Thomas' NHS Foundation Trust, London

Mr Leo Nherera, NCC-CC
Health Economist, Royal College of Physicians of London

Dr Stephen Rogers, Royal College of General Practitioners
Senior Lecturer in Primary Care, University College, London

Dr Peter Rose, invited as an expert in haematology to attend GDG meetings 3 and 4
Consultant Haematologist, South Warwickshire General Hospitals NHS Trust

Mr Peter Rose, The Stroke Association
Patient/Carer Representative, Information Service Organiser for the East of England, The Stroke Association

Mrs Fiona Sayers, Royal College of Nursing
Nurse Practitioner, Frimley Park Hospital NHS Foundation Trust, Surrey

Mr David Smith, British Cardiac Patients Association
Patient/Carer Representative, Trustee, British Cardiac Patients Association

Dr Neil Sulke, British Cardiac Society
Consultant Cardiologist, East Sussex Hospitals NHS Trust, Eastbourne

Preface

The association of an irregular pulse with morbidity has been recognised since antiquity, and as long ago as 1628 William Harvey observed cardiac irregularity directly in animals. The modern emphasis on electrical demonstration of atrial fibrillation (AF) dates back a mere 100 years to the first publication by William Einthoven of an electrocardiogram showing the abnormality. Even the treatment of this disorder has a long and venerable history: William Withering published *An account of the foxglove and some of its medical uses* in 1785, and digoxin, the active extract of his remedy, remains in use today.

A patient developing AF in 2006 is faced with a wide array of potential therapies. A number of drugs can be employed to control the rapid heart rate, which is often an intrinsic part of AF; attempts can be made to restore sinus rhythm using drugs or direct current electrical shock; and an increasing number of surgical procedures are described. Despite the wide number of options available, there is an acknowledgement that AF is too frequently treated with the almost automatic prescription of monotherapy with digoxin: this is still a useful drug over 200 years on but the best option for only a minority of patients. This failure to appreciate or implement proper treatment options in such a common condition makes AF an excellent topic for a national clinical guideline.

The guideline covers aspects of diagnosis and the management of AF in a number of different circumstances. It covers paroxysmal, persistent and permanent AF, considers AF developing after surgical procedures, and offers advice on haemodynamically unstable AF. Many of the recommendations relate to control of AF and the important decision of whether to attempt to restore sinus rhythm or concentrate on control of the heart rate. In a linked set of recommendations, the importance of considering anticoagulation in all these patients is emphasised. This is sometimes neglected in clinical practice, but anticoagulation is of enormous potential benefit because of its role in stroke prevention, and one of the key recommendations in the guideline is that the risk of thromboembolism should be formally assessed. A simple clinical model that includes advice on appropriate prophylaxis is suggested for this purpose. Other key recommendations cover the use of the electrocardiogram in diagnosis, and the preference in most patients for beta-blockers or rate-limiting calcium antagonists over digoxin for rate control.

The work of producing the guideline has been in the hands of a Guideline Development Group (GDG) comprising a small team from the National Collaborating Centre for Chronic Conditions working together with patients and health professionals with particular interest and experience in the management of AF. They have used the available evidence and their own clinical and personal judgement to produce guidance that is both clinically relevant and methodologically sound.

The GDG has had to evaluate a large amount of evidence during this process, and debate on some of the recommendations has been lively. The members have been driven throughout by the desire to produce a guideline that will be of value throughout the NHS. I am grateful to them for their hard work and for their expertise, and I am confident that they have produced a guideline that deserves to meet that aim.

Dr Bernard Higgins MD FRCP
Director, National Collaborating Centre for Chronic Conditions

List of abbreviations

AF	Atrial fibrillation
ARR	Absolute risk reduction
AV	Atrioventricular
AVJ	Atrioventricular junction (also called atrioventricular node)
bid	Twice daily
BSA	Body surface area
CABG	Coronary artery bypass graft
CHF	Congestive heart failure
CI	Confidence interval
Class Ic	Vaughan-Williams Class Ic antiarrhythmic drug
Class II	Vaughan-Williams Class II antiarrhythmic drug
Class III	Vaughan-Williams Class III antiarrhythmic drug
cm	Centimetre
CTR	Cardiothoracic ratio
CV	Cardioversion
CXR	Chest X-ray
DC	Direct current
ECG	Electrocardiogram
ECV	Electrical cardioversion
GDG	Guideline Development Group
Hg	Mercury
ICD	Implantable cardioverter defibrillator
ICER	Incremental cost-effectiveness ratio
ICH	Intracranial haemorrhage
INR	International normalised ratio
IV	Intravenous
LAA	Left atrial appendage
LAA-A	Left atrial appendage area
LAA-V	Left atrial appendage flow velocity
LAD	Left atrial diameter (synonymous with left-atrial dimension)
LA	Left atrium
LBBB	Left bundle branch block
LMWH	Low molecular weight heparin
LV	Left ventricular
LVEDD	Left ventricular end diastolic diameter
LVESD	Left ventricular end systolic diameter
LVEF	Left ventricular ejection fraction

LVFS	Left ventricular fractional shortening
LVH	Left ventricular hypertrophy
M	Metre
mg	Milligram
MI	Myocardial infarction
mm	Millimetre
mmol	Joule
N	Number of study participants
NCC-CC	National Collaborating Centre for Chronic Conditions
NICE	National Institute for Health and Clinical Excellence
NNT	Numbers needed to treat
NPV	Negative predictive value
NR	Not reported
NS	Not statistically significant
NSAID	Non-steroidal anti-inflammatory drug
NSF	National service framework
NYHA	New York Heart Association (functional classification)
OR	Odds ratio
p	Probability of a result happening by chance rather than because of a genuine effect
PCV	Pharmacological cardioversion
PPV	Positive predictive value
PVI	Pulmonary vein isolation
QALY	Quality-adjusted life-years
qid	Four times daily
RA	Right atrium
RAA	Right-atrial appendage
RBBB	Right bundle branch block
RCT	Randomised controlled trial
RR	Relative risk
sec	Second
SVT	Supraventricular tachycardia
TDP	Torsades des pointes
TEE	Thromboembolic event
TIA	Transient ischaemic attack
tid	Three times daily
TOE	Transoesophageal echocardiogram
TTE	Transthoracic echocardiogram
UK	United Kingdom
WMI	Wall motion index
WPW	Wolff–Parkinson–White syndrome

DEVELOPMENT OF THE GUIDELINE

1 | Introduction

1.1 Definition

Atrial fibrillation (AF) is an atrial tachyarrhythmia characterised by predominantly uncoordinated atrial activation with consequent deterioration of atrial mechanical function. Another closely related atrial arrhythmia is atrial flutter, and this will also be discussed in the guideline insofar as its treatment coincides with that of AF itself.

On the electrocardiogram, AF is described by the absence of consistent P waves; instead there are rapid oscillations or fibrillatory waves that vary in size, shape and timing and are generally associated with an irregular ventricular response when atrioventricular (AV) conduction is intact. The patient may experience AF as palpitations, chest pain, dizziness, or in extreme cases loss of consciousness. In many cases, however, it may occur asymptomatically.

The ventricular response in AF depends on many things, including AV nodal properties, the level of vagal and sympathetic tone and drugs that affect AV nodal conduction such as beta-blockers, non-dihydropyridine calcium-channel blockers (calcium antagonists) and digitalis glycosides. However, regular relative risk (RR) intervals on the electrocardiogram (ECG) may occur, for example, in the presence of heart block associated with conduction disease or drug therapy. In patients with permanent ventricular pacing, the diagnosis may require temporary pacemaker inhibition in order to visualise AF activity. A rapid, irregular, sustained, wide QRS complex tachycardia could suggest AF with conduction via an accessory pathway.

1.2 Classification

Recent guidelines suggest classification of AF based on the temporal pattern of the arrhythmia (see Table 1.1).

Table 1.1 Classification of AF subtypes

Terminology	Clinical features	Pattern
Initial event (first detected episode)	Symptomatic Asymptomatic (first detected) Onset unknown (first detected)	May or may not reoccur
Paroxysmal	Spontaneous termination <7 days and most often <48 hours	Recurrent
Persistent	Not self-terminating Lasting >7 days or prior cardioversion	Recurrent
Permanent ('Accepted')	Not terminated Terminated but relapsed No cardioversion attempt	Established

Table reprinted with permission from Levy S, Camm AJ, Saksena S et al. International consensus on nomenclature and classification of atrial fibrillation. *Europace* 2003;5:119–22.[1]

AF is considered *recurrent* when a patient experiences two or more episodes. These episodes may be paroxysmal if they terminate spontaneously, defined by consensus as 7 days, or persistent if the arrhythmia requires electrical or pharmacological cardioversion for termination. Successful termination of AF does not alter the classification of persistent AF in these patients.

Long-standing AF (defined as over a year) that is not successfully terminated by cardioversion, or when cardioversion is not pursued, is classified as permanent.

Paroxysmal AF, in which the frequency of paroxysms is low, may degenerate into either paroxysmal AF with more frequent paroxysms, or a sustained form of AF. Similarly, persistent AF may degenerate into permanent AF. Despite its name, the reversion of permanent AF to normal sinus rhythm is also possible, particularly in those cases where the AF is caused by an underlying disease process which is successfully treated (eg thyroid disease), or where a specialist procedure is performed that modifies the electrophysiological properties of the heart.

Without treatment, AF can sometimes result in a degree of haemodynamic instability which can represent a critical condition that requires immediate intervention to alleviate symptoms of breathlessness, chest pain and loss of consciousness, and restore haemodynamic stability.

1.3 Epidemiology

1.3.1 Prevalence

AF is the commonest sustained cardiac arrhythmia. Much of the epidemiology of AF is derived from data from predominantly white populations, and information on AF in non-white populations is scarce. Hospital practice data may give a biased view of the clinical epidemiology of AF, since only one-third of patients with AF may actually have been admitted to hospital.[2]

The prevalence of AF roughly doubles with each advancing decade of age, from 0.5% at age 50–59 years to almost 9% at age 80–89 years.[3] Conversely, AF is very uncommon in infants and children, unless concomitant structural or congenital heart disease is present.

In the UK, the Renfrew–Paisley study[4] found that of an original cohort of men and women aged 45–64 years (N=15,406) there were 100 (0.65%; 95% CI 0.53 to 0.79%) documented cases of AF. The prevalence of AF increased with age and more cases were detected in men (53 of 7,052) than women (47 of 8,354)[4] as shown in Figure 1.1. In the West Birmingham AF project, the prevalence of AF was 2.4% in two general practices[2] and further extension of this project showed that the prevalence of AF among Indo-Asians aged over 50 years in the general practice population was 0.6%.[5] The Newcastle survey screened 4,843 people aged 65 years or more in general practices and found a prevalence of AF of 4.7%.[6] Among UK hospital admissions, AF is present in 3–6% of acute medical admissions.[7,8]

The 4-year incidence of AF in the Renfrew–Paisley project was 0.54 cases per 1,000 person years[4] (see Figure 1.2).

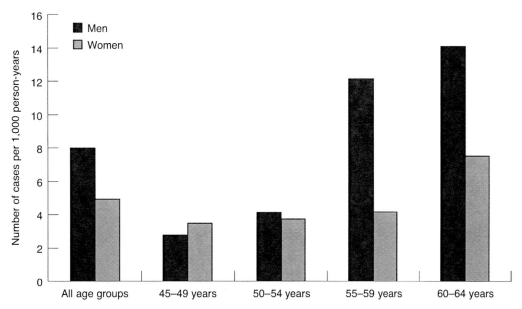

Figure 1.1 Prevalence of AF in the Renfrew–Paisley project.[4*]

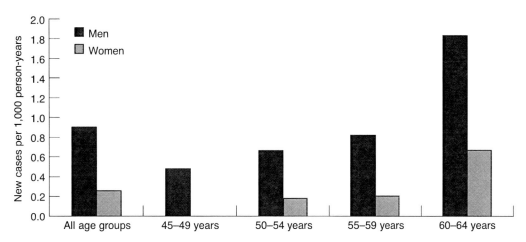

Figure 1.2 Incidence of AF in the Renfrew–Paisley project.[4] *Figures 1.1 and 1.2 were reproduced with permission of BMJ Publishing Ltd from Stewart S, Hart CL, Hole DJ et al. Population prevalence, incidence, and predictors of atrial fibrillation in the Renfrew/Paisley study. *Heart* (British Cardiac Society) 2001;86:516–21.

1.3.2 Risk factors

There are many risk factors for developing AF. As discussed above, there is an increasing prevalence and incidence of AF with increasing age. In the Framingham study[9] the development of AF was associated with increasing age (odds ratio (OR) 2.1 for men and 2.2 for women, p <0.0001), diabetes (OR 1.4 for men and 1.6 for women), hypertension (OR 1.5 for men and 1.4 for women), and valve disease (OR 1.8 for men and 3.4 for women). It is also commonly associated with, and complicated by, congestive heart failure and strokes.

AF is often caused by coexisting medical conditions. These causes can be cardiac and non-cardiac (see Table 1.2).

Table 1.2 Common cardiac and non-cardiac causes of AF	
Cardiac causes of AF	**Non-cardiac causes of AF**
Common cardiac causes: ischaemic heart disease rheumatic heart disease hypertension sick sinus syndrome pre-excitation syndromes (eg Wolff–Parkinson–White).	Acute infections, especially pneumonia
	Electrolyte depletion
	Lung carcinoma
Less common cardiac causes: cardiomyopathy or heart muscle disease pericardial disease (including effusion and constrictive pericarditis) atrial septal defect atrial myxoma.	Other intrathoracic pathology (eg pleural effusion)
	Pulmonary embolism
	Thyrotoxicosis

AF is also common after surgery, especially cardiothoracic operations such as thoracotomy and coronary artery bypass graft. Overall, the presence of the AF after surgery not only results in prolongation of hospital stay but may also increase risk of heart failure, stroke, or thromboembolism, and greater hospital costs. The incidence of postoperative AF depends on many risk factors apart from the type of procedure, such as age and the patient's preoperative physiology and electrolyte balance.

Many dietary and lifestyle factors have also been associated with AF. These include excessive alcohol or caffeine consumption and emotional or physical stress. In the case of alcohol, AF may develop as a consequence of an excessive intake of alcohol over a relatively short period – a so-called 'holiday heart'. In one series of younger patients (aged <65 years) with new onset AF, alcohol caused or contributed to the arrhythmia in 63% of cases.[10]

Lone AF is defined as AF without overt structural heart disease, and defined by a normal clinical history and examination, ECG, chest X-ray and, more recently, the echocardiogram. There are implications of labelling patients with this diagnosis, as this group is often considered to be at 'low risk', although recent data have been inconclusive.

A diagnosis of lone AF is only considered a diagnosis of exclusion if there is:
- no history of cardiovascular disease or hypertension
- no abnormal cardiac signs on physical examination
- a normal chest X-ray and, apart from the presence of AF, a normal ECG (ie no indication of prior myocardial infarction or left ventricular hypertrophy)
- normal atria, valves and left ventricular size and function by echocardiography.

1.4 Prognosis

The adverse effects of AF are the result of haemodynamic changes related to the rapid and/or irregular heart rhythm, and thromboembolic complications related to a prothrombotic state associated with the arrhythmia. AF is associated with an odds ratio for death of 1.5 for men and 1.9 in women, which does not vary by age, but most of the excess of mortality attributed to AF occurs early after diagnosis of AF.[11]

Onset of AF can result in a reduction in cardiac output of up to 10–20% regardless of ventricular rate. The presence of fast ventricular rates can push an already compromised ventricle into heart failure. An uncontrolled AF rate may even precipitate critical cardiac ischaemia.

AF is associated with a prothrombotic state – intra-atrial blood stasis, structural heart disease or blood vessel abnormalities and abnormal platelets and haemostasis – leading to a predisposition to thrombus formation (thrombogenesis).[12] This prothrombotic state predisposes to stroke and thromboembolism in AF, with an approximately five-fold greater risk than that of people without AF.[13] In stroke patients, concurrent AF is associated with greater disability, longer in-hospital patient stay and lower rate of discharge to own home. The incidence of strokes attributable to AF increases from 1.5% at age 50–59 years to 23.5% at age 80–89 years.[14]

In terms of the direct effects on patients' quality of life, AF can also result in reduced exercise tolerance, as well as impairment in cognitive function.

1.5 Guideline structure

Chapter 2 details the methodology used in the construction of this guideline. This includes the protocols used for the searching, selection and appraisal of evidence, and the grading of recommendations according to the strength of their supporting evidence.

The remaining chapters deal with specific issues in the diagnosis and treatment of AF. For ease of reference, wherever possible different forms of AF have been considered in distinct chapters, as follows:

- persistent AF (Chapter 6)
- permanent AF (Chapter 7)
- paroxysmal AF (Chapter 8)
- acute-onset AF (Chapter 9)
- postoperative AF (Chapter 10).

Most of these chapters include an easy-to-use flowchart showing the recommendations relevant to the particular form of AF.

There are also chapters dedicated to the identification and diagnosis of AF, as well as to antithrombotic therapy and cardioversion.

1.6   How to use this guideline

- The purpose of this guideline is to support clinical judgement, not to replace it. This means the treating clinician should:
  - take into consideration any contraindications in deciding whether or not to administer any treatment recommended by this guideline
  - consider the appropriateness of any recommended treatment for a particular patient in terms of the patient's relevant clinical and non-clinical characteristics.

- Wherever possible, before administering or changing any treatment the treating clinician should follow good practice in terms of:
  - discussing with the patient why the treatment is being offered and what health outcomes are anticipated
  - highlighting any possible adverse events or side effects that have been associated with the treatment
  - obtaining explicit consent for the treatment.

- For those recommendations involving pharmacological treatment, the most recent edition of the *British National Formulary* (**www.bnf.org.uk**) should be followed for the determination of:
  - indications
  - drug dosage
  - method and route of administration
  - contraindications
  - supervision and monitoring
  - product characteristics.

  Exceptions to the above are cases where guidance is provided within the recommendation itself.

- The guideline will normally only make drug recommendations that fall within licensed indications. If a drug is recommended outside of its licensed indication this will be made clear in the guideline (see Appendix D).

2 Methodology

2.1 About the guideline

2.1.1 Aim

With this document the National Collaborating Centre for Chronic Conditions (NCC-CC) has aimed to provide a user-friendly, clinical, evidence-based guideline for the National Health Service (NHS) in England and Wales that:

- offers best clinical advice for AF
- is based on best published evidence and expert consensus
- takes into account patient choice and informed decision-making
- defines the major components of NHS care provision for AF
- indicates areas suitable for clinical audit
- details areas of uncertainty or controversy requiring further research
- provides a choice of guideline versions for differing audiences.

2.1.2 Scope

The guideline was developed in accordance with a scope which detailed the remit of the guideline originating from the Department of Health and specified those aspects of AF to be included and excluded. Prior to the commencement of the guideline development, the scope was subjected to stakeholder consultation in accordance with processes established by the National Institute for Health and Clinical Excellence (NICE).[15] The full scope is shown in Appendix G.

This guideline sets out best practice for the diagnosis and treatment of AF in both primary and secondary care. It also considers which patients benefit from referral for specialist investigations or procedures and offers guidance in this respect.

Most of the recommendations made in this guideline apply to both AF and the closely related arrhythmia atrial flutter (in those cases where the two conditions are indistinguishable). Exceptions are recommendations concerning diagnosis and opportunistic case-detection, which apply only to AF.

Although the guideline covers the majority of AF cases, it does not consider those patients for whom there is a need for highly specialised clinical input. In particular, it does not consider paediatric cases of AF, or gestational AF.

With the exception of the use of prophylactic drugs to prevent postoperative AF and the use of typical symptoms in guiding opportunistic case-detection, the guideline will not consider issues of public health screening or interventions.

The guideline does not make any recommendations in terms of health service delivery for AF treatment, although it does consider the effectiveness of different service models. In particular, it considers the effectiveness of self-management of anticoagulation compared to clinic-based management, and the use of pill-in-the-pocket therapy compared with continuous drug therapy or emergency department treatment.

2.1.3 Audience

The guideline is intended for use by the following people or organisations:
- all healthcare professionals
- people with AF and their carers
- patient support groups
- commissioning organisations
- service providers.

2.1.4 Patient involvement

The NCC-CC was keen to ensure that the views and preferences of people with AF and their carers informed all stages of the guideline. This was achieved by:
- having a person with AF and a representative of a user organisation on the Guideline Development Group (GDG)
- consulting the Patient Information Unit (PIU) housed within NICE during the pre-development (scoping) and final validation stages of the guideline.

2.1.5 Guideline limitations

Limitations to the guideline are as follows:
- Clinical guidelines usually do not cover issues of service delivery, organisation or provision (unless specified in the remit from the Department of Health).
- NICE is primarily concerned with health services and so recommendations are not provided for social services and the voluntary sector. However, the guideline may address important issues in how NHS clinicians interface with these other sectors.
- Generally the guideline does not cover rare, complex, complicated or unusual conditions.

2.2 Guideline development

2.2.1 Background

The development of this evidence-based clinical guideline draws upon the methods described by the NICE *Guideline development methods* manual[16] (**www.nice.org.uk/page.aspx?o=201982**) and the methodology pack[17] specifically developed by the National Collaborating Centre for Chronic Conditions (NCC-CC) for each chronic condition guideline (**www.rcplondon.ac.uk/college/ceeu/ncccc_index.htm**). The developers' roles and remit are summarised below.

▷ National Collaborating Centre for Chronic Conditions

The NCC-CC was set up in 2001 and is housed within the Royal College of Physicians. The NCC-CC undertakes commissions received from the National Institute for Health and Clinical Excellence (NICE).

A multiprofessional partners' board inclusive of patient groups and NHS management governs the NCC-CC.

▷ NCC-CC technical team

The technical team met approximately two weeks before each GDG meeting and comprised:
- the GDG group leader
- the GDG clinical advisor
- an information scientist
- a research fellow
- a health economist
- a project manager
- administrative personnel.

▷ Guideline Development Group[16]

The GDG met 14 times between July 2004 and December 2005 and comprised a multidisciplinary team of professionals, service users (people with AF or carers), and user organisation representatives who were supported by the technical team.

The GDG membership details, including patient representation and professional groups, are listed at the front of this guideline (see pages vi–vii).

Members of the GDG declared any interests in accordance with the NICE technical manual.[16] A register is available from the NCC-CC for inspection upon request (ncc-cc@rcplondon.ac.uk).

▷ Sign-off workshop[17]

At the end of the guideline development process the GDG met to review and agree the guideline recommendations.

2.2.2 The guideline development process

There are ten basic steps in the process of producing a guideline.

▷ Step 1: Developing evidence-based questions

The technical team drafted a series of clinical questions that covered the guideline scope. The GDG and Project Executive refined and approved these questions, shown in Appendix C.

▷ Step 2: Systematically searching for the evidence

The information scientist developed a search strategy for each question. Key words for the search were identified by the GDG. In addition, the health economist searched for additional papers to inform detailed health economic work (eg modelling). Papers that were published or accepted for publication in peer-reviewed journals were considered as evidence by the GDG. Conference paper abstracts and non-English language papers were excluded from the searches.

Each clinical question dictated the appropriate study design that was prioritised in the search strategy but the strategy was not limited solely to these study types. The research fellow or health economist identified titles and abstracts from the search results that appeared to be relevant to the question. Exclusion lists were generated for each question together with the rationale for the exclusion. The exclusion lists were presented to the GDG. Full papers were obtained where relevant. See Appendix C for literature search details.

▷ Step 3: Critically appraising the evidence

The research fellow or health economist, as appropriate, critically appraised the full papers. In general no formal contact was made with authors but there were *ad hoc* occasions when this was required in order to clarify specific details. Critical appraisal checklists were compiled for each full paper. One research fellow undertook the critical appraisal and data extraction. The evidence was considered carefully by the GDG for accuracy and completeness.

All procedures are fully compliant with:
- NICE methodology as detailed in the *Guideline development methods – information for National Collaborating Centres and guideline developers* manual.[16]
- NCC-CC quality assurance document and systematic review chart, available at **www.rcplondon.ac.uk/college/ceeu/ncccc_index.htm**

▷ Step 4: Incorporating health economic evidence

There were constraints in the health economic resources and so the following approach was agreed for this guideline. Health economics was incorporated alongside the clinical questions.
- Searches in relevant databases were done by the information scientist using economic filters on the related clinical questions.
- No study design criteria were imposed a priori, ie the searches were not limited to randomised control trials (RCTs) or formal economic evaluations.
- Titles and abstracts identified in the economic searches were reviewed by the health economist and full papers were obtained once they met the inclusion/exclusion criteria.
- The full papers were critically appraised by the health economist and the relevant data were presented to the GDG.

Cost-effectiveness evidence from the UK was preferred, but all relevant evidence was considered, including non-UK studies.

The GDG identified areas for additional economic work. Five key areas were identified and three were given priority. The GDG agreed on the model structures. The health economist performed supplemental literature searches using key search terms in Medline and an Internet search engine to obtain additional information for modelling. None of the identified priority areas were modelled for various reasons (see Appendix A for details).

▷ Step 5: Distilling and synthesising the evidence and developing recommendations

The evidence from each full paper was distilled into an evidence table and synthesised into evidence statements before being presented to the GDG. This evidence was then reviewed by the GDG and used as a basis upon which to formulate recommendations.[2]

▷ Step 6: Grading the evidence statements and recommendations

The criteria for grading evidence and classifying recommendations are shown in Table 2.1.

Evidence tables are available at
www.rcplondon.ac.uk/pubs/online_home.htm

Table 2.1 Criteria for grading evidence and recommendations. Note that diagnostic study levels of evidence and classification of recommendations were also included.[16]

Levels of evidence		Classification of recommendations	
Level	Type of evidence	Class	Evidence
1++	High-quality meta-analysis (MA), systematic reviews (SR) of randomised controlled trials (RCTs), or RCTs with a very low risk of bias.	A	Level 1++ and directly applicable to the target population or level 1+ and directly applicable to the target population AND consistency of results. Evidence from NICE technology appraisal.
1+	Well-conducted MA, SR or RCTs, or RCTs with a low risk of bias.		
1–	MA, SR of RCTs, or RCTs with a high risk of bias.	Not used as a basis for making a recommendation.	
2++	High-quality SR of case-control or cohort studies. High-quality case-control or cohort studies with a very low risk of confounding, bias or chance and a high probability that the relationship is causal.	B	Level 2++, directly applicable to the target population and demonstrating overall consistency of results. or extrapolated evidence from 1++ or 1+.
2+	Well-conducted case-control or cohort studies with a low risk of confounding, bias or chance and a moderate probability that the relationship is causal.		
2–	Case-control or cohort studies with a high risk of confounding, bias or chance and a significant risk that the relationship is not causal	Not used as a basis for making a recommendation.	
3	Non-analytic studies (for example case reports, case series).	C	Level 2+, directly applicable to the target population and demonstrating overall consistency of results or extrapolated evidence from 2++.
4	Expert opinion, formal consensus.	D	Level 3 or 4 or extrapolated from 2+ or formal consensus.
		D (GPP)	A good practice point (GPP) is a recommendation based on the experience of the GDG.

Diagnostic study level of evidence and classification of recommendation was also included.[2]

13

▷ Step 7: Agreeing the recommendations

The sign-off workshop employed formal consensus techniques to:
- ensure that the recommendations reflected the evidence base
- approve recommendations based on lesser evidence or extrapolations from other situations
- reach consensus recommendations where the evidence was inadequate
- debate areas of disagreement and finalise recommendations.

The sign-off workshop also reached agreement on the following:
- five priorities for implementation
- five key research recommendations
- algorithms.

In prioritising key recommendations for implementation, the sign-off workshop also took into account the following criteria:
- high clinical impact
- high impact on reducing variation
- more efficient use of NHS resources
- allowing the patient to reach critical points in the care pathway more quickly.

The audit criteria provide suggestions of areas for audit in line with the key recommendations for implementation.[16]

▷ Step 8: Structure of the guideline

The guideline is divided into sections for ease of reading. For most sections the layout is similar and is described below:
- The *clinical introduction* sets a succinct background and describes the current clinical context.
- The *methodological introduction* describes any issues or limitations that were apparent when reading the evidence base.
- *Evidence statements* provide a synthesis of the evidence base and usually describe what the evidence showed in relation to the outcomes of interest.
- *Health economics* presents, where appropriate, an overview of the cost effectiveness of the evidence base.
- *From evidence to recommendations* highlights the debate of the GDG. This section sets out the GDG decision-making rationale providing a clear and explicit audit trail from the evidence to the evolution of the recommendations.
- The *recommendations* section provides stand-alone, action-orientated recommendations.
- *Evidence tables* are not published as part of the full guideline but are available online at **www.rcplondon.ac.uk/pubs/books/af/** These describe comprehensive details of the primary evidence that was considered during the writing of each section.

▷ Step 9: Writing the guideline

The first draft version of the guideline was drawn up by the technical team in accordance with the decision of the GDG. The guideline was then submitted for two formal rounds of public and stakeholder consultation prior to publication.[16] The registered stakeholders for this guideline are detailed in Appendix F. Editorial responsibility for the full guideline rests with the GDG.

Table 2.2 describes the versions of the guideline that are available.

Table 2.2 Versions of this guideline	
Full version	Details the recommendations. The supporting evidence base and the expert considerations of the GDG. Available at **www.rcplondon.ac.uk/pubs/online_home.htm**
NICE version	Documents the recommendations without any supporting evidence. Available at **www.nice.org.uk/page.aspx?o=guidelines.completed**
Quick reference guide	An abridged version. Available at **www.nice.org.uk/page.aspx?o=guidelines.completed**
Information for the public	A lay version of the guideline recommendations. Available at **www.nice.org.uk/page.aspx?o=guidelines.completed**

▷ Step 10: Updating the guideline

Literature searches were repeated for all of the evidence-based questions at the end of the GDG development process allowing any relevant papers published up until 30 June 2006 to be considered. Future guideline updates will consider evidence published after this cut-off date.

Two years after publication of the guideline, NICE will commission a National Collaborating Centre to determine whether the evidence base has progressed significantly to alter the guideline recommendations and warrant an early update. If not, the guideline will be updated approximately 4 years after publication.[16]

2.3 Disclaimer

Healthcare providers need to use clinical judgement, knowledge and expertise when deciding whether it is appropriate to apply guidelines. The recommendations cited here are a guide and may not be appropriate for use in all situations. The decision to adopt any of the recommendations cited here must be made by the practitioner in light of individual patient circumstances, the wishes of the patient, clinical expertise and resources.

The NCC-CC disclaims any responsibility for damages arising out of the use or non-use of these guidelines and the literature used in support of these guidelines.

2.4 Funding

The National Collaborating Centre for Chronic Conditions was commissioned by the National Institute for Health and Clinical Excellence to undertake the work on this guideline.

3 | Key messages of the guideline

3.1 Priorities for implementation

The following five recommendations have been identified by the GDG as priorities for implementation:

1. An electrocardiogram (ECG) should be performed in all patients, whether symptomatic or not, in whom AF is suspected because an irregular pulse has been detected.

2. As some patients with persistent AF will satisfy criteria for either an initial rate-control or rhythm-control strategy (for example, aged over 65 but also symptomatic):
   - the indications for each option should not be regarded as mutually exclusive and the potential advantages and disadvantages of each strategy should be explained to patients before agreeing which to adopt
   - any comorbidities that might indicate one approach rather than the other should be taken into account
   - irrespective of whether a rate-control or a rhythm-control strategy is adopted in patients with persistent AF, appropriate antithrombotic therapy should be used.

3. In patients with permanent AF, who need treatment for rate control:
   - beta-blockers or rate-limiting calcium antagonists should be the preferred initial monotherapy in all patients
   - digoxin should only be considered as monotherapy in predominately sedentary patients.

4. In patients with newly diagnosed AF for whom antithrombotic therapy is indicated (see section 11.6), such treatment should be initiated with minimal delay after the appropriate management of comorbidities.

5. The stroke risk stratification algorithm (Figure 11.1) should be used in patients with AF to assess their risk of stroke and thromboembolism, and appropriate thromboprophylaxis given.

Each of these recommendations highlights areas of current clinical practice that the GDG believe would particularly benefit from guidance. Compliance with each of these key priority areas may be audited according to the corresponding audit criteria below.

Although items 4 and 5 may be audited using the same criteria, they address two different issues relating to antithrombotic therapy in AF. The first addresses the need for appropriate anti-thrombotic therapy in patients with AF upon initial diagnosis; the second addresses the need for a formal assessment of stroke risk and the administration of appropriate antithrombotic therapy based on that assessment.

3.2 AF care pathway

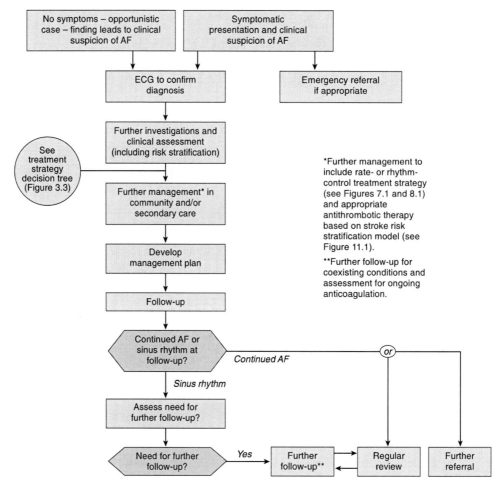

Figure 3.1 AF care pathway

3.3 Treatment strategy decision tree

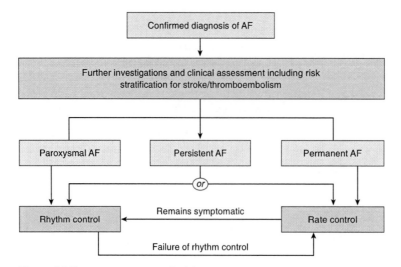

Figure 3.2 Treatment strategy decision tree

3.4   Audit criteria

Table 3.1 lists the audit criteria identified to evaluate the impact of the implementation of the five key priority areas detailed above on clinical practice and health outcomes.

Table 3.1 Audit criteria for the key priorities for implementation		
Criterion	**Exception**	**Definition of terms**
1. All people presenting to primary or secondary care with a history of hypertension, heart failure, diabetes or stroke and noted to have an irregular pulse to be offered an ECG and any new diagnosis of AF recorded.	None.	Percentage of patient records with a new diagnosis of AF made following an ECG made on the basis of detection of an irregular pulse.
2. All AF patients in whom a rate-control or rhythm-control strategy is initiated to have their involvement in choosing a treatment strategy recorded.	Postoperative or haemodynamically unstable patients, or those otherwise not able to engage in a decision-making process.	Percentage of patient records with a record of involvement of the patient in the decision-making process.
3. All patients who are prescribed digoxin as initial monotherapy for rate control to have the reason for this prescription recorded where it is not obvious (eg sedentary patient, presence of contraindication to alternative agents).	None.	Percentage of patient records with a prescription of digoxin for initial rate-control monotherapy where the reason for digoxin prescription is: • sedentary patient • presence of contra-indications to beta-blockers or rate-limiting calcium antagonists • other reasons.
4 and 5. All patients should be assessed for risk of stroke/ thromboembolism and given thromboprophylaxis according to the stroke risk stratification algorithm (see Figure 11.1) and have this assessment and any antithrombotic therapy recorded.	Haemodynamically unstable patients or those in whom assessment is impossible or inappropriate.	Percentage of patient records with a record of risk assessment and thromboprophylaxis consistent with the stroke risk stratification algorithm.

Note: numbers correspond to the numbered list of key priorities for implementation.

3.5   Areas for future research

The GDG has identified the following five questions as key areas for further research:

▷   Cardioversion

Although cardioversion is a core treatment for many patients with AF, there is little evidence that compares the different modes (electrical and pharmacological), particularly in terms of cost effectiveness. Further, the studies that have considered the efficacy of preloading with antiarrhythmic drugs prior to electrical cardioversion have not reported long-term efficacy in maintaining sinus rhythm, or the cost effectiveness of this strategy.

- In patients scheduled for elective cardioversion what is the optimal form of cardioversion, in terms of the pre-cardioversion use of antiarrhythmic drugs, the mode of cardioversion (electrical or pharmacological), the cost effectiveness of each procedure and the impact on quality of life?

▷   Echocardiography

Echocardiography allows cardiac abnormalities such as left ventricular impairment to be diagnosed earlier than would be possible from signs and symptoms alone. However, no study has addressed the issue of whether performing routine echocardiography on all newly diagnosed AF patients would be more cost effective in diagnosing and treating heart disease earlier, than performing echocardiography only on those patients in whom there is a clinical suspicion of undiagnosed heart disease.

- What is the cost effectiveness of performing a routine echocardiographic examination in all newly diagnosed AF patients, compared to only selective examination based on clinical criteria?

▷   Anticoagulation with antiplatelet therapy

In the general AF population, the evidence suggests that combined therapeutic anticoagulation with antiplatelet therapy does not reduce the incidence of stroke or thromboembolism compared with therapeutic anticoagulation alone, and it may increase the incidence of bleeding. However, it is unclear whether there are certain subgroups of patients with AF for whom the therapeutic effects of combination therapy may be greater than either monotherapy. In particular, it is unclear whether combination therapy is justified in those AF patients who have stent implantation or a history of myocardial infarction (MI).

- Is there any additional benefit, in terms of overall vascular events, from combined anticoagulation with antiplatelet therapy for any subgroups of patients with AF such as those with prior MI or stent implantation?

▷   Pill-in-the-pocket treatment

Some patients with paroxysmal AF may have paroxysms infrequently. In these patients, the continuous use of antiarrhythmic drugs to suppress paroxysms may not be justified relative to their toxicity. No study has been undertaken in such patients in a UK population to determine whether a pill-in-the-pocket treatment strategy would be clinically or cost effective compared with either the emergency department administration of treatment or continuous antiarrhythmic drug therapy.

- What is the clinical and cost effectiveness of pill-in-the-pocket treatment for those with paroxysmal AF compared with hospital-based administration or continuous antiarrhythmic therapy?

▷ Anticoagulation in paroxysmal AF

The frequency of paroxysms in patients with paroxysmal AF varies widely between patients. It remains unclear, however, whether the risk of stroke or thromboembolism varies between those with only infrequent paroxysms and those with more frequent paroxysms. It is also unclear whether, if the risk of stroke or thromboembolism is reduced in those with infrequent paroxysms, the use of anticoagulation is justified in such a low-risk group.

- What is the optimal anticoagulation strategy for those patients with paroxysmal AF who have infrequent paroxysms, and those who have more frequent paroxysms?

THE GUIDELINE

4 Identification and diagnosis

4.1 Presenting symptoms/pulse palpitation

AF can present in the setting of a wide variety of cardiac and non-cardiac conditions, it is often asymptomatic and can present with vague non-specific symptoms. Too often, AF is only detected after the patient presents with serious complications of AF, such as a stroke, thromboembolism or heart failure. The initial diagnosis of AF depends on associating symptoms such as breathlessness, dyspnoea, palpitations, syncope/dizziness or chest discomfort with AF.

Most of the data on presentation of AF patients have been based on white Caucasian populations, and limited data are available in relation to ethnicity and AF.[18] Furthermore, there may be important differences between hospital-based cohorts compared with community or population-based studies, as many do not present to hospital care, and if they do, it is often in the context of associated comorbidity such as ischaemic heart disease or heart failure. Indeed, many patients with AF in general practice remain asymptomatic. However, as AF commonly occurs in association with risk factors, such as hypertension, diabetes and ischaemic heart disease, opportunistic assessment of such patients for the presence of AF may be prudent, especially since such patients are frequently seen for check-ups in primary care.

While general population screening is beyond the scope of this guideline, targeted/opportunistic screening of symptomatic patients or those with risk factors may allow identification of AF patients. One recent study[19,20] aims to determine the baseline prevalence and the incidence of AF based on a variety of screening strategies and in doing so to evaluate the incremental cost effectiveness of different screening strategies, including targeted or whole population screening, compared with routine clinical practice, for detection of AF in people aged 65 and over. This study[20] – whose publication date fell outside of the date limits of the systematic literature search – reported that the baseline prevalence of AF in subjects older than 65 was 7.2%, with a higher prevalence in men (7.8%) and among patients aged 75 or older (10.3%), and indicated that the only strategy that improved on routine practice was opportunistic screening.

4.1.1 Methodological introduction

The results of nine studies are included in this report. Seven studies were critically appraised.[7,8,21–25] Of these, none reported the frequency of presenting symptoms in primary care in a UK (or other) population. Patients presenting to secondary care generally present with more severe symptoms. The studies:

- did not use a consistent terminology to classify AF symptoms. 'Dizziness' was also referred to as 'near syncope'[21] and 'chest pain' was also referred to as 'chest discomfort'[22]
- were single-centre studies
- had a variable proportion of patients presenting with *de novo* AF versus those with a previous history of AF.

Three of the appraised studies were not based on UK populations.[21–23] One study[8] reported the frequency of presenting symptoms between ethnic groups (white, Asian and black groups) but the numbers were too small to perform statistical comparisons.

4.1.2   Evidence statements

Dyspnoea, chest pain and palpitations were found to be the most common presenting symptoms in emergency admissions with newly diagnosed or previously diagnosed AF in the UK[7,8] or USA.[26-28]

Table 4.1 Presenting symptoms associated with emergency AF admissions					
Study	N	Dyspnoea %	Chest pain %	Palpitations %	Dizziness /syncope %
Zarifis et al[8]	245	47.1	19.9	16.2	16.2
Lip et al[7]	170	51.8	34.1	25.9	18.8
Michael et al[26]	289	7	10	78	3
Burton et al[27]	266	12	24	40	9

Similar results were found in patients with chronic[23] (more than 7 days since onset of symptoms) and lone AF.[21]

In one study[24] (N=756) dyspnoea was the most commonly reported symptom in chronic and recent-onset AF (46.8%); palpitations were the most commonly reported symptom in paroxysmal AF (79.0%).[28]

Table 4.2 Presenting symptoms between paroxysmal, chronic and recent-onset AF patients				
Symptom	Total	Paroxysmal	Chronic	Recent-onset
Palpitations (%)	54.1	79	44.7	51.5
Chest pain (%)	10.1	13.2	8.2	11
Dyspnoea (%)	44.4	22.8	46.8	58
Syncope/dizziness (%)	10.4	17.4	8	9.5
Fatigue (%)	14.3	12.6	13.1	18
Other (%)	0.9	0	1.8	0
None (%)	11.4	5.4	16.2	7

In two studies, stroke was reported as a presenting symptom of AF at rates of 5.1% and 3.2% respectively[22,25] and occurred at a rate of 12.7% in a study population combining both new-onset and previously diagnosed AF.[8,28]

4.1.3   From evidence to recommendations

Those with undiagnosed AF can receive treatment sooner if an opportunistic case finding is undertaken using manual pulse palpation in those presenting with symptoms commonly associated with AF. It was therefore considered good practice to check the blood pressure and pulse (manually) in all patients who present with breathlessness, dyspnoea, palpitations, syncope/dizziness or chest discomfort.

Many patients presenting with stroke are also found to be in AF, indicating a missed opportunity to diagnose the pre-existing AF and administer appropriate antithrombotic therapy.

RECOMMENDATION

R1   In patients presenting with any of the following:
- breathlessness/dyspnoea
- palpitations
- syncope/dizziness
- chest discomfort
- stroke/TIA

manual pulse palpation should be performed to assess for the presence of an irregular pulse that may indicate underlying AF.   C

4.2   Electrocardiography

As with many chronic disorders, AF may be symptomatic or asymptomatic, and episodes of either can occur in the same patient.

Most symptomatic patients with AF present with symptoms related to the arrhythmia. However, such patients can have a wide variety of other cardio-respiratory presenting symptoms and clinical features[7,24] (see section 4.1).

Many patients with AF are asymptomatic and are picked up in general practice. One study[2] found that a third of AF patients had not had hospital contact for symptoms related to AF. Asymptomatic AF can be discovered incidentally during clinical examination by cardiac auscultation, 12-lead ECG recording, or 24-hour Holter recording that may have been performed for unrelated reasons.

The patient may also have presented with associated medical problems, such as heart failure, stroke or thromboembolism, and coincidental AF is detected. The duration of AF may be unknown in such patients, and whether AF was the cause or effect of the acute problem (eg stroke or heart failure) may be uncertain.

Many patients with risk factors for developing AF, such as hypertension and diabetes, do attend regular checkups with their GPs. In these cases then, there is the possibility of opportunistic case finding.

4.2.1 Methodological introduction

The two studies performed in UK primary care[29,30] evaluated the finding of an irregular pulse as a screening test for AF. Both studies included populations of over 65-year-olds and confirmed the diagnosis of AF by ECG.

4.2.2 Evidence statements

In one study,[29] the diagnostic accuracy of pulse palpation was compared between different age and gender groups in a primary care population aged 65 or over, and is summarised in Table 4.3. (II)

Table 4.3 Diagnostic accuracy of pulse palpitation between different age and gender groups				
	Women 75+	Women 65–74	Men 75+	Men 65–74
Sensitivity	93 (66 to 100)	100 (16 to 100)	95 (75 to 100)	100 (54 to 100)
Specificity	71 (66 to 77)	86 (81 to 91)	71 (65 to 77)	79 (74 to 84)
PPV	14 (7 to 22)	8 (1 to 25)	23 (14 to 34)	12 (4 to 23)
NPV	99 (97 to 100)	100 (98 to 100)	99 (96 to 100)	100 (98 to 100)

All values are percentages with 95% confidence intervals.

One study[30] measured the diagnostic accuracy of three different methods of nurse-based screening for AF based on the presence of either continuous or intermittent pulse irregularities over a minimum of 20 seconds in a population aged over 65. The results are as shown in Table 4.4. (II)

Table 4.4 Comparison of the diagnostic accuracy of three different methods of pulse palpation to screen for the presence of AF			
	Method 1	Method 2	Method 3
Sensitivity	91 (82 to 97)	72 (59 to 82)	54 (41 to 66)
Specificity	74 (72 to 77)	94 (93 to 96)	98 (97 to 99)
PPV	19 (15 to 23)	44 (35 to 54)	61 (47 to 73)
NPV	99 (98 to 100)	98 (97 to 99)	97 (96 to 98)

All values are percentages with 95% confidence intervals. Method 1: diagnostic accuracy based on the detection of any pulse irregularity; method 2: diagnostic accuracy based on the detection of frequent or continuous irregularities; method 3: diagnostic accuracy based on the detection of only continuous irregularities.

4.2.3 From evidence to recommendations

An irregular pulse was found to be sensitive to the presence of AF.[29] The positive predictive value was greater in those over 75 years old, as the prevalence of AF is known to be higher in this population. The negative predictive value of a regular pulse (>96%) was also emphasised. The results of a second study[30] suggested it would be prudent to consider any pulse irregularity as requiring further investigation to determine whether AF is present.

One study[19,20] whose publication date fell outside of the date limits of the systematic literature search confirmed the above results in an elderly UK population (over 65 years old). The study also showed that opportunistic case-detection for AF is a more cost-effective strategy than systematic screening and is associated with fewer ischaemic strokes and a greater proportion of diagnosed AF cases.

The evidence did not consider clinical indicators other than an irregular pulse and it was agreed that where there were other clinical indicators suggestive of AF, an ECG should still be performed. Nonetheless, the majority of patients presenting with AF will have an irregular pulse that may occur in the absence of any symptoms, and it is unlikely that AF will be present if the pulse is normal.

The diagnosis of AF does not require a 12-lead ECG recording. In the case of atrial flutter, however, a 12-lead ECG may be necessary, and may also occur in the presence of a regular pulse. The recommendation made below therefore applies only to AF case detection.

RECOMMENDATION

R2   An electrocardiogram (ECG) should be performed in all patients, whether symptomatic or not, in whom AF is suspected because an irregular pulse has been detected.   B(DS)

4.3   Ambulatory ECG recording

Many patients with intermittent AF have asymptomatic paroxysms. In one study[31] it was estimated that only 1 in 12 paroxysms are symptomatic. Nonetheless, these patients remain at risk of complications associated with AF.

In patients with daily paroxysms, clinical practice is to perform a 24-hour Holter monitor, but this is less useful in patients who get paroxysms at intervals of more than 24 hours. In the latter category of patients, event ECGs (including transtelephonic monitors ('cardiomemos') and some implanted systems) are commonly used to detect/diagnose AF.

4.3.1   Methodological introduction

Ambulatory-ECG was defined as any electrocardiographic recording device that continuously recorded cardiac electrical activity while the patient was able to move around relatively freely without hindrance. Ambulatory-ECG included both Holter-monitoring and implanted recorders such as programmed pacemakers that generated a continuous ECG recording.

Event-ECG was defined as any electrocardiographic recording device which recorded only particular events, identified either automatically by a software program to detect arrhythmic episodes or by the onset of symptoms (when the patient manually switches on the device for the duration of the symptomatic episode), or a combination of the two. As with ambulatory-ECGs, event-ECGs record cardiac electrical activity while the patient is able to move around relatively freely without hindrance.

Studies were included if the sample population was reported to be patients with either suspected AF or suspected atrial arrhythmia. No studies compared the diagnostic accuracy of event-ECG devices with ambulatory-ECG devices over the same duration.

4.3.2 Evidence statements

One cross-over study[32] of patients suspected of atrial arrhythmia based on palpitations compared a patient-triggered event recorder over a mean period of 70 hours with a 48-hour Holter monitor. The event recorder detected proportionately more symptomatic episodes than the Holter monitor (67% of recorded episodes associated with symptoms versus 35% respectively; p<0.001) **(1b)**. Similarly, the event recorder yielded more arrhythmia diagnoses (19% versus 0% respectively; p<0.005). **(1b)**

In one study[33] which compared 24-hour Holter monitoring with automatic and patient triggered event recording (each over 30 days), the automatically-triggered event recorder had a higher diagnostic yield than the patient-triggered event recorder, which in turn had a higher diagnostic yield for diagnoses of AF than the Holter monitor (24%, 13% and 5% respectively). The automatically triggered event recorder was also more effective than the patient-triggered event recorder in detecting asymptomatic episodes of AF (52 events versus 1 event respectively).[34]

In one study[35] of 139 patients admitted with symptoms of acute stroke or transient ischaemic attack (TIA) who were ECG-negative for AF/flutter, seven (5%) were picked up in a second round of monitoring using a 24-hour Holter monitor. A further five (6%) patients were diagnosed with AF/flutter in a third round of monitoring using a 7-day event recorder (with both patient and automated triggering).[34]

4.3.3 From evidence to recommendations

No studies were found to compare the positive diagnostic yield per unit time between an ambulatory-ECG diagnostic tool and an event-ECG tool where the recordings were interpreted in a comparable manner.

One study[35] found that the use of event-ECG detected cases of AF remained undetected by both non-ambulatory and ambulatory-ECG. In addition, the study found that the use of ambulatory-ECG detected cases of AF remained undetected by non-ambulatory-ECG.

Also, a strategy of event-ECG diagnosis detected more symptomatic episodes and more positive diagnoses of atrial arrhythmias, including AF, than the strategy of ambulatory-ECG diagnosis.

RECOMMENDATION

R3   In patients with suspected paroxysmal AF undetected by standard ECG recording:

-   a 24-hour ambulatory ECG monitor should be used in those with suspected asymptomatic episodes or symptomatic episodes less than 24 hours apart
-   an event recorder ECG should be used in those with symptomatic episodes more than 24 hours apart.   B(DS)

4.4   Echocardiography

Although most cardiologists will perform a transthoracic echocardiogram (TTE) on patients with AF referred to cardiology clinics,[36] echocardiography is not undertaken on all patients seen in primary or non-specialist secondary care.[2,7,8,37]

Regarding the use of echocardiography to identify stroke risk factors, although most stroke risk stratification criteria (see Appendix A) lay emphasis on clinical risk factors, there is a perception that TTE is mandatory to decide on antithrombotic therapy. In one study[38] echocardiography revealed cardiac abnormalities in many AF patients, although most had other clinical risk factors for thromboembolism and often echocardiography did not alter the management decision.

In clinical practice echocardiography has also been used to assess the risk of recurrent AF post cardioversion, as well as to assess the risk of developing postoperative AF. Finally, transoesophageal echocardiography (TOE) has been used to guide cardioversion (TOE-guided cardioversion (see section 5.4)), but this is a specialist investigation. TOE can also be used by specialists to assess the risk of stroke and thromboembolism.[39]

4.4.1   Methodological introduction

The results of 29 studies were included in this report. Studies were considered for inclusion if echocardiographic (TTE or TOE) variables were stratified into normal and abnormal ranges and tested, alongside clinical variables, as independent risk factors for clinically defined outcomes.

The clinical outcomes considered were:
-   AF pathophysiology
-   the recurrence of AF following successful cardioversion
-   stroke or thromboembolism
-   vascular death.

The presence of intracardiac thrombus was not considered as an echocardiographic measure of structural or functional heart disease. Rather, it was considered as a consequence of the disease.

4.4.2   Evidence statements

▷   AF pathophysiology

One study[40] found a left atrial diameter greater than 50 mm to be the only significant independent echocardiographic predictor for the development of a greater AF burden, in terms of the amount of time spent in AF or the frequency of AF episodes ($p < 0.05$). (2++)

One study[41] found that in patients developing AF, it is more likely to lead to haemodynamic instability in patients with an atrial filling fraction less than 40% (RR 2.7; p<0.0001), or left-ventricular dysfunction (p<0.03) during sinus rhythm. (2+)

▷ Post-cardioversion recurrence

Left atrial haemodynamic dysfunction, as measured by a left atrial appendage velocity (LAA-V) greater than 40 cm/sec, has been found to be a significant independent predictor of maintained sinus rhythm following cardioversion in one study[42] (OR 5.2, 95% CI 2.7 to 10; p<0.0001). In another study,[43] a ratio of left atrial appendage area (LAA-V) over the left atrial area (LA area) greater than 0.009 was found to be an independent predictor of maintained sinus rhythm (OR 6.4; 95% CI 1.9 to 2.4; p=0.004). (2+)

Left atrial haemodynamic dysfunction, as measured by the presence of spontaneous echo contrast (SEC) in the left atrium, has not been found to be an independent predictor of sinus rhythm maintenance following cardioversion.[42,44] (2++)

Based on the results of four studies,[42,45–47] left atrial diameter is not an independent predictor of sinus rhythm maintenance following cardioversion (2+). However, two studies[44,48] did find a left atrial diameter of less than 45 mm (p=0.02) or less than 41 mm (p=0.008) to be an independent predictor. (2++)

One study,[45] while not finding left atrial diameter to be an independent predictor of sinus rhythm maintenance following cardioversion, did find a right atrial diameter of less than 37 mm to be an independent predictor (OR 5.9; 95% CI 1.4 to 25; p<0.02). (2+)

The presence of moderate or severe heart failure (NYHA>1) has been found to be an independent predictor of AF recurrence following cardioversion in one study[49] (p<0.0005) (2++). Another study,[46] found no such relationship between left ventricular dysfunction, when measured as either left ventricular end diastolic diameter (LVEDD) or left ventricular end systolic diameter (LVESD), and sinus rhythm maintenance. (2+)

One study[42] did not find the presence of mitral regurgitation to be an independent predictor AF recurrence following cardioversion (2+). Another study[50] found the presence of mitral annular abnormalities to be able to effectively predict the recurrence of AF at 12 months following cardioversion (positive predictive value (PPV) 79%, negative predictive value (NPV) 85%). (2+)

▷ Stroke or thromboembolism

Two studies[51,52] did not find aortic stenosis to be an independent predictor of stroke or thromboembolism. (2+)

One study[53] found the presence of complex aortic plaque to be an independent predictor of stroke in those over 70 years (OR 4.0, 95% CI 1.1 to 14; p=0.03). The same study did not find the same result in those under 70. (2++)

Based on the results of four studies,[51,53–55] it is unclear whether left atrial haemodynamic dysfunction, as measured by the presence of SEC, is an independent predictor of stroke or thromboembolism. (2++)

Based on the results of two studies,[55,56] left atrial haemodynamic dysfunction, as measured by LAA-V less than 20 cm/sec, is an independent predictor of stroke or thromboembolism (2+). Another study[53] found a similar result in those under 70 years, but not in those over 70 years. (2++)

Based on the results of six studies,[52,54,57–60] it is unclear whether an enlarged left atrium, measured either in terms of area or diameter, is an independent predictor of stroke or thromboembolism. (2+)

Based on the results of three studies,[57,61,62] (echocardiographically detected) left ventricular dysfunction is an independent predictor of stroke or thromboembolism: (2++)
- $RR = 2.5$ (1.5 to 4.4), $p<0.001$[61]
- $RR = 2.6$ (1.4 to 4.9), $p=0.003$[57]
- $OR = 1.8$ (1.2 to 2.7), $p=0.003$.[62]

Two other studies[51,54] did not find left ventricular dysfunction to be an independent predictor. (2+)

Based on the results of two studies,[52,62] left ventricular hypertrophy is an independent predictor of stroke or thromboembolism: (2+)
- $OR = 2.8$ (1.8 to 4.4), $p=0.0001$[62]
- $OR = 6.56$, $p<0.01$.[52]

Another study[51] did not find left ventricular hypertrophy to be an independent predictor. (2+)

Two studies[51,52] did not find mitral annular calcification to be an independent predictor of stroke or thromboembolism. (2+)

A meta-analysis of three clinical trials[61] (N=1,066) failed to find either mitral valve prolapse or regurgitation (of any degree) to be independent predictors of stroke or thromboembolism (2++). However, the results of a smaller study (N=290)[59] suggested that moderate-to-severe mitral regurgitation may be an independent negative predictor of stroke (OR 0.45, 95% CI 0.20 to 0.97) in a population at a low risk of stroke. (2++)

▷ Vascular death

One study[63] found that left-atrial haemodynamic dysfunction, as indicated by spontaneous echo contrast, was an independent predictor of vascular death in patients with AF, defined as either fatal non-haemorrhagic stroke, MI, congestive heart failure (CHF), systemic embolism or sudden cardiac death syndrome (RR 7.96, 95% CI 1.6 to 41; $p=0.013$) (2++). The study did not find the presence of structural, valvular or aortic cardiovascular disease to be independent predictors. (2++)

4.4.3 From evidence to recommendations

Echocardiography is able to identify factors that are independently predictive of successfully maintaining sinus rhythm following cardioversion. In particular, LAA-V measured by TOE is able to independently predict the successful maintenance of sinus rhythm following cardio-version.[42,43] TOE may therefore be used, in addition to other clinical variables, in determining the appropriateness of pursuing a rhythm-control strategy involving cardioversion.

In most cases risk stratification for stroke or thromboembolism and the decision to administer appropriate thromboprophylaxis can be made on purely clinical (non-echocardiographic) characteristics. However, the stroke risk may be unclear in some patients, in which case echocardiography may be useful in refining the risk. In particular, TOE may be used to identify the presence of complex aortic plaque[53] and impaired left atrial haemodynamics.[53,55,56] TTE may be used to identify left ventricular dysfunction or hypertrophy,[57,61,62] that may not be associated with overt heart failure.[52,62]

In many patients with AF, there may be indications other than the AF itself that make it necessary to perform an echocardiographic examination. For example, it may be used to identify suspected co-present heart disease. TOE may further be used to detect cardiac abnormalities not identified through TTE (eg patent foramen ovale).

The recommendations made here are specifically for those instances where echocardiography is used in relation to AF and how the results may influence the choice of treatment strategy or antiarrhythmic drug.

RECOMMENDATIONS

R4   Transthoracic echocardiography (TTE) should be performed in patients with AF:
- for whom a baseline echocardiogram is important for long-term management, such as younger patients   D(GPP)
- for whom a rhythm-control strategy that includes cardioversion (electrical or pharmacological) is being considered   C
- in whom there is a high risk or a suspicion of underlying structural/functional heart disease (such as heart failure or heart murmur) that influences their subsequent management (for example, choice of antiarrhythmic drug)   D(GPP)
- in whom refinement of clinical risk stratification for antithrombotic therapy is needed (see section 11.6).   C

R5   TTE should not be routinely performed solely for the purpose of further stroke risk stratification in patients with AF for whom the need to initiate anticoagulation therapy has already been agreed on appropriate clinical criteria (see section 11.6).   D(GPP)

R6   Transoesophageal echocardiography (TOE) should be performed in patients with AF:
- when TTE demonstrates an abnormality (such as valvular heart disease) that warrants further specific assessment   D(GPP)
- in whom TTE is technically difficult and/or of questionable quality and where there is a need to exclude cardiac abnormalities   D(GPP)
- for whom TOE-guided cardioversion is being considered.   D(GPP)

5 Cardioversion

5.1 Electrical versus pharmacological cardioversion

Cardioversion is performed as part of a rhythm-control treatment strategy, and if successful restores sinus rhythm.[64] However, not all attempts at cardioversion are successful, and at one year post cardioversion approximately 50% of patients are back in AF.[65]

There are two types of cardioversion: electrical (ECV) and pharmacological (PCV). The optimal techniques and recommended protocols for performing cardioversion have been widely discussed in the literature.[64,66–68] PCV involves the use of various antiarrhythmic drugs, some of which may also be used to maintain sinus rhythm after electrical cardioversion (see section 6.1) or concomitantly with ECV (see section 5.3). Current clinical practice regards PCV as the preferred strategy in patients presenting with AF of recent onset (within 48 hours); ECV is regarded as the preferred strategy where the AF is more prolonged. Cardioversion is not normally attempted until possible underlying precipitants (eg thyrotoxicosis, infections) have been successfully treated and any electrolyte abnormalities corrected.

In clinical practice, young patients who develop AF but have no underlying structural heart disease often have an acute identifiable precipitant for their AF (eg alcohol). These cases often revert spontaneously to sinus rhythm without the need to attempt cardioversion (ECV or PCV).

5.1.1 Methodological introduction

Two studies were used to measure the success and failure rates of cardioversion but neither used double blinding and they may have been subject to expectation bias or confounding. Both studies had short follow-up periods, and therefore the incidence of thromboembolism or longer-term adverse events were not reliably measured. Neither study considered outcome measures such as exercise capacity or overall quality of life. There were conflicting results for the outcome measure 'duration of hospital stay', so no reliable conclusions could be drawn regarding health economic outcome measures.

5.1.2 Evidence statements

No difference has been found in rates of successful cardioversion between ECV and PCV as the initial treatment strategy (73% versus 74% respectively,[69] and 77% versus 81% respectively[70]). (1+)

Patients who had PCV as the initial treatment option, followed by ECV if sinus rhythm was not restored, were more likely to be cardioverted than those patients in whom the treatment preference was reversed (96% versus 84% respectively; $p<0.05$)[69] (1+). Similar results were observed for a subgroup of patients with lone AF (100% versus 77% $p<0.01$) although no significant differences have been found for those with either chronic or recent-onset AF or those with structural heart disease.[69] (1+)

Initiating treatment with PCV cost less per successful cardioversion than initiating treatment with ECV in all patients (US$1,240 versus US$1,917 p=0.002).[69] Initial PCV also cost less per successful cardioversion in patients with lone AF (US$965 versus US$2,021), and in patients with structural heart disease (US$1,223 versus US$1,814). Mean cost per patient was US$1,188 in the initial PCV and US$1,603 in the initial ECV group. The increased cost of ECV was attributed to heart monitoring, medications and oxygen.

5.1.3 From evidence to recommendations

Few studies set out to compare which patients would benefit most from ECV versus PCV. Two studies[69,70] failed to find any difference between these strategies when used as the initial treatment option. Concern was expressed regarding the overall applicability of the results of one study[70] to UK clinical practice. The health economics data supported the clinical outcomes that using PCV as first-line treatment followed by ECV if PCV failed was the most cost effective. The health economic study costings were based on US dollars.

The evidence failed to address many issues (eg incidence of thromboembolism and stroke, and improvements to quality of life). The choice of strategy was considered to be dependent on local facilities and available expertise. It was recognised that some clinicians perform elective cardioversion under general anaesthesia, while others performed the procedure under sedation. Also, there has been a move towards nurse-led cardioversion services.[71–73]

As the treatments were considered equally effective, highlighting patient choice was important. Informing patients that neither treatment has been shown to be more effective than the other is important and can help to prevent patients becoming disillusioned when cardioversion fails.

It was concluded that the available evidence suggested pharmacological and electrical cardioversion to be of comparable efficacy in recent onset AF. However, it was felt that in more prolonged cases of AF electrical cardioversion is the preferred option based on clinical experience and current clinical practice. It was also felt preferable to attempt cardioversion as soon as possible following AF onset to maximise the likelihood of a successful outcome.

RECOMMENDATION

R7 In patients with AF without haemodynamic instability for whom cardioversion is indicated:
- the advantages and disadvantages of both pharmacological and electrical cardioversion should be discussed with patients before initiating treatment   D(GPP)
- where AF onset was within 48 hours previously, either pharmacological or electrical cardioversion should be performed   B
- for those with more prolonged AF (onset more than 48 hours previously) electrical cardioversion should be the preferred initial treatment option.   D(GPP)

5.2　Pharmacological cardioversion

Clinical practice commonly uses Vaughan-Williams Class Ia, Ic and III antiarrhythmic drugs for PCV.[68] However, these agents are associated with a risk of proarrhythmia in the presence of electrolyte abnormalities and ischaemic or structural heart disease.[74–76] This risk should be considered when choosing drugs for individual patients. The fast-acting intravenous beta-blocker esmolol has also been used and shown to be effective.[77,78] Digoxin has been shown to be ineffective for use in PCV.[79–81]

Patients undergoing PCV are usually admitted to hospital and have the antiarrhythmic drug administered intravenously, under ECG monitoring. These drugs may also be administered orally, and have been shown to have comparable efficacy to intravenous administration at 24 hours.[82–85] On occasion, an oral antiarrhythmic agent may be prescribed for those patients with paroxysmal AF where the drug has previously been known to work effectively and safely, and there are no contraindications (see section 8.2).

In the UK, the most commonly used drugs for PCV in patients with persistent AF are amiodarone, flecainide, propafenone and sotalol. This section addresses the efficacy of amiodarone versus the other three drugs.

5.2.1　Methodological introduction

The results of 15 studies are reported; one was a meta-analysis,[86] and the remainder were RCTs.

The meta-analysis[86] compared the efficacy of amiodarone to the Class Ic agents flecainide or propafenone, but did not report the individual drug comparisons separately. The results of two studies[85,87] included in the meta-analysis were not reported separately, one[85] because a statistical comparison was not made between the study drugs, and the other[87] because the study was only available in Italian.

All of the studies considered the comparison between two intravenously or orally administered antiarrhythmic drugs. Studies comparing the oral administration of one drug with the intravenous administration of another were excluded on the basis that the route of administration could confound the results of drug efficacy.

Regarding the comparison between the two Class III agents, amiodarone and sotalol, only one study[88] compared intravenous amiodarone with intravenous sotalol, but with additional oral administration of each drug as required. Although not licensed in the UK, results involving the intravenous preparation of propafenone have been included in this report as conclusions may be extrapolated to flecainide (as an intravenous flecainide preparation is licensed in the UK), or to oral preparations of propafenone.

With one exception,[89] all of the studies were in patients with acute- or recent-onset AF (in all cases less than 2 weeks). However, in three studies[88,90,91] only patients with acute-onset of less than 24 or 48 hours were considered. All studies excluded patients with moderate-to-severe heart failure (New York Heart Association (NYHA) grade greater than II) or left ventricular dysfunction. All studies reported the restoration of sinus rhythm as primary outcome, rather than the frequency of side effects associated with each drug.

5.2.2 Evidence statements

▷ Amiodarone versus sotalol

One study[88] reported no significant difference in efficacy between an intravenous/oral combination of amiodarone and sotalol for the restoration of sinus rhythm in patients with AF or atrial flutter of less than a 24-hour duration (1+). A similar result was reported in another study[89] using only oral administration, where both drugs were administered prior to electrical cardioversion. (1++)

One study[88] reported no significant difference in the frequency of adverse side effects between amiodarone and sotalol for the cardioversion of acute-onset AF or atrial flutter (two instances of heart failure in the amiodarone-treated group – both of which occurred in patients with impaired left ventricular function (LVEF) <40% – versus two instances of hypotension in the sotalol-treated group). (1+)

▷ Amiodarone versus flecainide/propafenone

A meta-analysis[86] of seven primary studies comparing parenteral or oral formulations of amiodarone with either flecainide or propafenone, found flecainide/propafenone to be more effective than amiodarone in restoring sinus rhythm within the first 8 hours after administration, but not at 24 hours (see Table 5.1). (1+)

Table 5.1 Relative risk of remaining in AF with flecainide or propafenone compared with amiodarone over different time periods	
Time (hours)	RR (95% CI)
2	0.35 (0.24 to 0.50)
5	0.44 (0.31 to 0.61)
8	0.57 (0.57 (sic.) to 0.80)
24	0.95 (0.83 to 1.09)

▷ Amiodarone versus flecainide

One study[90] (N=100) found intravenous flecainide to be more effective in terms of restoring sinus rhythm than intravenous amiodarone throughout the follow-up period of 12 hours, as well as in terms of the median time taken to restore sinus rhythm (1+). The results of another smaller study[92] did not find any significant difference throughout a follow-up period of 8 hours. (1+)

▷ Amiodarone versus propafenone

Three studies[90,91,93] found intravenous propafenone to be more effective and faster in restoring sinus rhythm than intravenous amiodarone for up to 8 hours following drug administration (1+). At 24 hours, the two drugs were comparable.[91,93] (1+)

One study[94] found no significant difference between propafenone and amiodarone in terms of restoring sinus rhythm when effectively administered as a single oral dose (with additional oral doses if sinus rhythm was not restored within 24 hours. (1+)

▷ Flecainide versus propafenone

Based on the results of four studies,[90,95–97] it is inconclusive whether intravenous flecainide is more effective than intravenous propafenone (see Table 5.2). (1+)

Table 5.2 Percentage of study participants reverting to sinus rhythm following administration of flecainide or propafenone					
Study	N	Time (hours)	Flecainide	Propafenone	p
Martinez-Marcos et al[90]	100	1	58	60	NS
Kingma et al[97]	70	1	86	55	<0.002
Kondili et al[96]	40	1	50	25	NS
Martinez-Marcos et al[90]	100	8	82	68	NS
Martinez-Marcos et al[90]	100	12	90	72	0.022

Three studies[90,95,96] found no significant difference in the mean time taken to restore sinus rhythm between intravenous flecainide and intravenous propafenone. (1+)

Based on the results of two studies, propafenone and flecainide are comparable in their efficacy[85,98] and speed[85] in restoring sinus rhythm when administered orally. (1+)

5.2.3 From evidence to recommendations

The evidence relied heavily on one study[90] with a relatively small number of patients (N=100). The evidence suggested that Class Ic drugs (flecainide and propafenone) are more effective than amiodarone at cardioverting patients with recent-onset AF at 2, 5, and 8 hours after administration. However, at 24 hours the difference in efficacy disappears, indicating that amiodarone has a longer period of onset than the Class Ic drugs. This result is also consistent with all of the primary studies, with no study finding any significant difference in efficacy at 24 hours or longer periods of observation.

The results of one study[90] suggested that flecainide and propafenone are comparable in terms of the time taken to revert to sinus rhythm (ie cardioversion), although at 12 hours flecainide was associated with a greater likelihood of reversion to sinus rhythm than propafenone was. A separate, unblinded study[88] suggested that for use in pharmacological cardioversion amiodarone and sotalol were comparable to each other in terms of both efficacy and safety.

It was noted that the trials excluded patients with structural or functional heart disease (left ventricular dysfunction). There were concerns about the use of Class I and Class III anti-arrhythmic drugs in these patients, although amiodarone was considered to be safe. The evidence assessing the use of digoxin for PCV was excluded from the literature search as this was considered to be an inappropriate use of this drug.

RECOMMENDATION

R8   In patients with persistent AF, where the decision to perform pharmacological cardioversion using an intravenous antiarrhythmic agent has been made:

- in the absence of structural heart disease,* a Class 1c drug (such as flecainide or propafenone) should be the drug of choice   B

- in the presence of structural heart disease,* amiodarone should be the drug of choice.   D(GPP)

*Coronary artery disease or left ventricular dysfunction.

5.3 Electrical cardioversion with concomitant antiarrhythmic drugs

Electrical cardioversion (ECV) alone is not always successful in inducing or maintaining sinus rhythm. In some cases, there is complete failure of ECV ('complete shock failure' or 'no conversion'). In other cases, AF recurs within a few minutes after a short period of sinus rhythm (immediate recurrence), sometimes recurrence is delayed from 1 day to 2 weeks (subacute or early recurrence), and sometimes AF recurrence occurs beyond 2 weeks (late recurrence).[99]

It is estimated that complete shock failure and immediate recurrence occur in approximately 25% of patients undergoing ECV, and subacute/early recurrences occur within 2 weeks in another 25%.[99]

In clinical practice, patients who have had a failed ECV or PCV or a relapse to AF while maintained on antiarrhythmic drugs, often have a further attempt at cardioversion, normally using ECV.

It is perceived that the concomitant administration of antiarrhythmic drugs increases the likelihood of successful cardioversion and the maintenance of sinus rhythm post cardioversion; this section addresses the evidence for this.

5.3.1 Methodological introduction

All 11 studies were RCTs, comparing either an antiarrhythmic drug with placebo[100–104] or comparing two or more antiarrhythmic drugs.[105,105–110] The results focus on the efficacy of concomitant antiarrhythmic drugs in ECV as none of the studies had sufficient power to detect differences in side effects.

Many of the studies considered the administration of antiarrhythmic drugs in both the pre-cardioversion and post-cardioversion periods. It is also unclear in many studies whether adjunctive rate-control therapy, such as digoxin or beta-blockers, was being prescribed in addition to the antiarrhythmic drugs.

The studies were similar in terms of patient population, drug dosages and outcome measures. There was some variance in the classification of successful cardioversion, as well as the policy on the inclusion or exclusion of patients with spontaneous cardioversion occurring prior to elective cardioversion.

5.3.2 Evidence statements

▷ Restoration of sinus rhythm

Four studies[101,105–107] compared pre-cardioversion amiodarone to rate-control drugs or placebo in relation to the incidence of successful cardioversion (see Table 5.3).

Table 5.3 Comparison of amidarone with various controls in terms of the incidence of successful cardioversion

	Study	N	Control	Amiodarone (%)	Control (%)	p
(1+)	Villani et al[105]	74	Digoxin	91	67	<0.05
(1+)	Villani et al[105]	90	Diltiazem	91	76	<0.05
(1+)	Capucci et al[107]	61	Diltiazem	87	65	<0.05
(1++)	Channer et al[101]	161	Placebo	72	79	NS
(1+)	Jong et al[106]	77	Various*	87	58	<0.05

*Study used either verapamil or propranolol to control ventricular rate.

One study[89] found that, in terms of the proportion of patients in whom sinus rhythm was restored either spontaneously or through the administration of electrical cardioversion, amiodarone and sotalol had equal efficacy (p=0.98) when administered from 28 days prior to scheduled cardioversion (1++). The study also found that those receiving either amiodarone or sotalol in the 28-day period prior to scheduled cardioversion had a higher prevalence of sinus rhythm at the end of the period, either through spontaneous restoration of sinus rhythm or through the administration of electrical cardioversion (p=0.01). (1++)

Six studies[100,102–105,108] compared various other antiarrhythmic drugs pre-cardioversion to rate-control drugs or placebo in relation to successful cardioversion (see Table 5.4).

Table 5.4 Comparison of various antiarrhythmic drugs with various controls in terms of the incidence of successful cardioversion

	Test/control	N	Test (%)	Control (%)	p
(1+)	Diltiazem/digoxin[105]	76	67	76	NS
(1++)	Flecainide/placebo[100]	54	73	82	NS
(1+)	Procainamide/placebo[104]	100	83	78	NS
(1+)	Propafenone/placebo[102]	35	73	74	NS
(1+)	Propafenone/placebo[103]	100	84.4	82.4	NS
(1+)	Verapamil/digoxin[108]	100	67	89	<0.05

One study[100] found pre-cardioversion flecainide use resulted in more successful first shocks in comparison with placebo (65% versus 30%, respectively; p=0.04). (1++)

▷ Recurrence of AF

The administration of amiodarone throughout the pre- and post-cardioversion period is associated with a reduced rate of relapse to AF compared with placebo or other drugs with a primary chronotropic effect (see Table 5.5).

Table 5.5 Comparison of amiodarone with other drugs or placebo in terms of the incidence of late AF recurrence post cardioversion

	Study	N	Control	Period (months)	Amiodarone (%)	Control (%)	p
(1+)	Villani et al[105]	74	Digoxin	1	28	78	<0.01
(1+)	Villani et al[105]	90	Diltiazem	1	28	56	<0.01
(1+)	Capucci et al[107]	61	Diltiazem	2	31	52	<0.01
(1++)	Channer et al[101]	161	Placebo	2	34	80	<0.001
(1+)	Jong et al[106]	77	Various*	2	37	77	<0.05

*Verapamil or propranolol.

It is unclear whether the administration of antiarrhythmic drugs pre-cardioversion decreases the likelihood of AF recurrence either in the first 48 hours following successful cardioversion or at up to 12 weeks (see Table 5.6).

Table 5.6 Comparison of antiarrhythmic drugs with control drugs in terms of the incidence of early or late AF recurrence post cardioversion

	Test/Control	N	Period	Test (%)	Control (%)	p
(1+)	Amiodarone/diltiazem[107]	61	24 hours	5	10	NS
(1+)	Amiodarone/digoxin[105]	74	24 hours	3	12	<0.01
(1+)	Diltiazem/digoxin[105]	76	24 hours	12	2	<0.01
(1+)	Amiodarone/diltiazem[105]	90	24 hours	3	2	NS
(1+)	Propafenone/placebo[103]	100	48 hours	12.2	35.8	<0.05
(1++)	Flecainide/placebo[100]	54	4 weeks	55	52	NS
(1+)	Verapamil/digoxin[108]	100	8 weeks	84	63	0.03
(1+)	Verapamil/digoxin[108]	100	12 weeks	91	72	0.03

One study[109] found the addition of verapamil to propafenone to be more effective than propafenone alone in terms of the incidence of post-cardioversion AF recurrence at 1 week and 3 months (1+). Another study[110] found no significant difference in the incidence of post-cardioversion AF recurrence at 1 week or 1 month between verapamil in addition to amiodarone and amiodarone alone. (1+)

▷ Defibrillation energy

It is inconclusive whether the administration of antiarrhythmic drugs is associated with either a reduced mean amount of energy per successful shock[102,104,105] or the total amount of energy per successful cardioversion attempt.[100,101,103,106] (1++)

5.3.3 From evidence to recommendations

Amiodarone and sotalol generally increased the likelihood of a successful cardioversion in comparison with controls in trials.[89,105–107] The historical literature regarding the amount of energy delivered during ECV was not considered to reflect current practice. These studies administered a low energy level shock and then escalated to a higher energy level shock. Therefore it was unclear whether the administration of antiarrhythmic drugs decreased the energy requirement for successful cardioversion. Furthermore, biphasic defibrillators (which deliver lower energy shocks) are increasingly used.

The evidence was also confounded by:

● the same antiarrhythmic drugs either being administered following a successful cardioversion for the long-term maintenance of sinus rhythm,[111,112] or

● the use of pre-cardioversion loading of antiarrhythmics not being reported in trial protocols, or considered as a comparison in long-term follow-up studies of sinus rhythm maintenance.

Measuring the immediate recurrence of AF was of limited value compared with recurrences in the longer term. From the limited data available based on small patient numbers, there was support for the use of amiodarone, sotalol and, possibly, propafenone in reducing the incidence of AF recurrences post cardioversion.

None of the evidence reflected concerns regarding potential adverse effects of antiarrhythmic drugs such as amiodarone. It was therefore not considered appropriate to recommend its use for routine ECV, although it may be beneficial in cases with a perceived increased risk of unsuccessful electrical cardioversion (eg long duration of AF).

There was no evidence found to support the use of other antiarrthymic drugs. Further, the concomitant use of digoxin did not improve cardioversion success.

RECOMMENDATION

R9   When patients with AF are to undergo elective electrical cardioversion and there is cause for heightened concern about successfully restoring sinus rhythm (such as previous failure to cardiovert or early recurrence of AF), concomitant amiodarone or sotalol* should be given for at least 4 weeks before the cardioversion.   B

*Sotalol to be progressively titrated from 80 mg twice daily up to 240 mg twice daily.

5.4 Transoesophageal echocardiography-guided cardioversion

Cardioversion of AF is associated with an increased risk of stroke and thromboembolism. In order to minimise this risk, anticoagulation is conventionally recommended for a minimum of 3 weeks before and during cardioversion, and for a minimum of 4 weeks after cardioversion. Even when pre-cardioversion transoesphageal echocardiography (TOE) fails to demonstrate left atrial thrombus, some patients have a thromboembolism post cardioversion (especially if no anticoagulation has been administered).[68,113]

As it may take some time to achieve therapeutic international normalised ratio for 3 consecutive weeks, some patients may wait months before cardioversion is attempted. As it is perceived that patients are more likely to successfully cardiovert the shorter the time they have been in AF, strategies to facilitate early cardioversion have been explored.

One strategy is TOE-guided cardioversion, where a patient with AF of more than 48 hours duration has a TOE to assess for intracardiac thrombus. In the absence of thrombus, heparin is usually given and cardioversion is performed. Anticoagulation with warfarin is subsequently continued for a minimum of 4 weeks. Patients in whom a thrombus is identified by TOE are considered at high risk of post-cardioversion thromboembolism and are usually treated with conventional therapeutic anticoagulation for at least 3 to 4 weeks before the TOE is repeated (see Figure 5.1). This strategy requires an experienced TOE operator, especially since visualisation of thrombus may be operator-dependent.

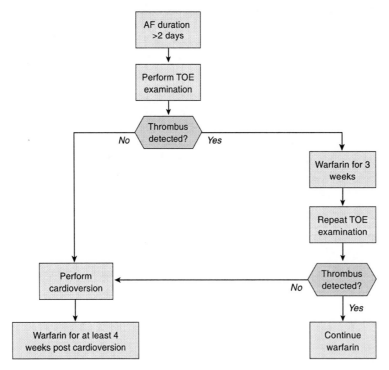

Figure 5.1 Cardioversion with TOE-guided strategy

5.4.1 Methodological introduction

Only studies where a comparison was made between a strategy of TOE-guided cardioversion and cardioversion without a prior TOE were included.

The primary clinical outcome of these studies was that the incidence of post-cardioversion thromboembolic events and other outcomes reported included the restoration and maintenance of sinus rhythm.

Of the two studies considering clinical outcomes included, one was a RCT,[114] and the other a cohort study.[115] In the former, in addition to the use of TOE examination, both the duration of anticoagulation and treatment were different between the two groups; in the later study, only the use of TOE examination was different between the two groups. Neither of the studies were adequately powered.

Of the two studies considering health economic outcomes,[116,117] one[117] estimated the cost per quality-adjusted life-year (QALY) of three strategies:
(1) conventional therapy transthoracic echocardiography (TTE) and warfarin therapy for one month before cardioversion)
(2) initial transthoracic echocardiography followed by transoesophageal echocardiographic-guided cardioversion and early cardioversion if no thrombus is detected (TTE/TOE)
(3) initial TOE-guided cardioversion with early cardioversion if no thrombus is detected.

The other study[116] estimated the costs and incremental cost per QALY of TOE-guided anticoagulation versus conventional anticoagulation based on the Assessment of Cardioversion Using Transoesophageal Echocardiography (ACUTE) trial.[114]

5.4.2 Evidence statements

One study[114] did not find any significant difference between TOE-guided cardioversion and a conventional strategy in terms of the incidence of thromboembolic events, stroke, successful initial cardioversion or maintenance of sinus rhythm at 8 weeks (1+). The difference in terms of mortality was of borderline significance (p=0.06) in favour of the conventional strategy. (1+)

A second study also failed to find any significant effect on the incidence of all embolic events between the two strategies.[115] (2+)

One study[114] found a lower incidence of bleeding events with a TOE-guided strategy compared with a conventional strategy (2.9% versus 5.5%, respectively; p=0.03). (1+)

TOE-guided cardioversion (US$ 2,774) costs less than TTE/TOE-guided cardioversion (US$3,070) and conventional strategy (US$3,106). Including the gains in QALYs, TOE-guided cardioversion is the least costly strategy with similar effectiveness (TOE accumulated 8.49 QALYs, TTE/TOE and conventional therapy both accumulated 8.48). The sensitivity analysis indicated that the results depend on a lower risk of cardioversion-related thromboembolism after negative TOE compared with conventional therapy.[117]

Overall, there was no significant difference in the mean costs per patient between TOE-guided and conventional care in the simulation model (US$3,503.09 versus US$3,423.52) and the hospital charge data from the ACUTE trial data (US$6,508 versus US$6,239, p=0.50). The analytic model indicated the initial treatment costs per patient were higher in the TOE group

(US$2,639.67 versus US$2,429.01), but outcome-associated costs were lower (US$863.42 versus US$994.51). The decision model indicated that the TOE-guided strategy costs US$185 more than conventional therapy when all treatment and outcome data are included (US$7,090 versus US$6,905). An incremental cost per QALY of TOE-guided cardioversion was calculated at US$15,455.[116]

5.4.3 From evidence to recommendations

Overall, the clinical studies suggest that TOE-guided cardioversion is of comparable efficacy to conventional strategy.[114,115] Although bleeding was reduced in the TOE-guided strategy, this was perceived to be a result of the shorter time spent on anticoagulation, and therefore TOE-guided cardioversion could be deemed preferable in patients with an increased bleeding risk. The health economic studies suggested that TOE-guided cardioversion may be a cost-effective treatment strategy.

The theoretical advantage of early cardioversion being more likely to be successful was not supported by the current clinical trial data. However, the studies were underpowered to detect significant differences in this, and in mortality and embolic event rates. TOE-guided cardioversion was considered a specialised procedure requiring appropriately experienced staff and appropriate facilities. However, it was considered that TOE-guided cardioversion should be an available treatment, as some patients would prefer the option of not being on prolonged anticoagulation.

RECOMMENDATION

R10 In patients with AF of greater than 48 hours duration, in whom elective cardioversion is indicated:

- both TOE-guided cardioversion and conventional cardioversion should be considered equally effective   B
- a TOE-guided cardioversion strategy should be considered:
    - where experienced staff and appropriate facilities are available, and   D(GPP)
    - where a minimal period of pre-cardioversion anticoagulation is indicated due to patient choice or bleeding risks.   C

5.5 Cardioversion treatment algorithm

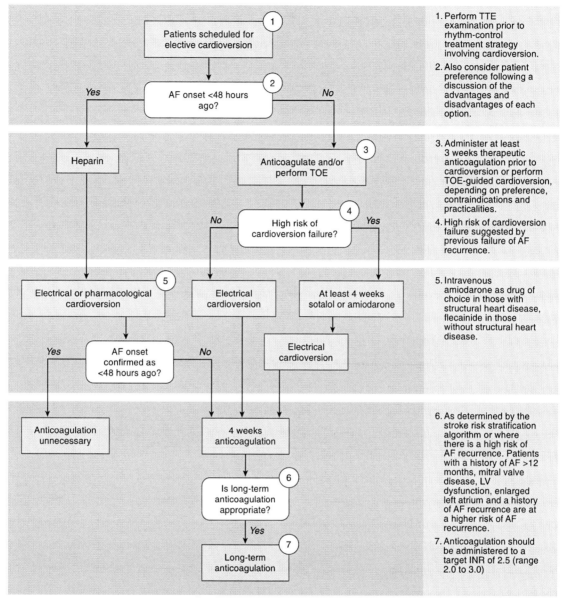

Figure 5.2 Cardioversion treatment algorithm

The diagram contents:

Patients scheduled for elective cardioversion (1)

AF onset <48 hours ago? (2)
- Yes → Heparin
- No → Anticoagulate and/or perform TOE (3)

High risk of cardioversion failure? (4)
- No → Electrical cardioversion
- Yes → At least 4 weeks sotalol or amiodarone → Electrical cardioversion

Heparin → Electrical or pharmacological cardioversion (5)

AF onset confirmed as <48 hours ago?
- Yes → Anticoagulation unnecessary
- No → 4 weeks anticoagulation

Is long-term anticoagulation appropriate? (6)
- Yes → Long-term anticoagulation (7)

Side notes:

1. Perform TTE examination prior to rhythm-control treatment strategy involving cardioversion.

2. Also consider patient preference following a discussion of the advantages and disadvantages of each option.

3. Administer at least 3 weeks therapeutic anticoagulation prior to cardioversion or perform TOE-guided cardioversion, depending on preference, contraindications and practicalities.

4. High risk of cardioversion failure suggested by previous failure of AF recurrence.

5. Intravenous amiodarone as drug of choice in those with structural heart disease, flecainide in those without structural heart disease.

6. As determined by the stroke risk stratification algorithm or where there is a high risk of AF recurrence. Patients with a history of AF >12 months, mitral valve disease, LV dysfunction, enlarged left atrium and a history of AF recurrence are at a higher risk of AF recurrence.

7. Anticoagulation should be administered to a target INR of 2.5 (range 2.0 to 3.0)

47

6 Treatment for persistent AF

6.1 Rate control versus rhythm control

AF is associated with increased mortality and morbidity. Currently, there are two main treatment strategies, rate control and rhythm control.

Rate control involves the use of chronotropic drugs or electrophysiological/surgical interventions to reduce the rapid heart rate (ventricular rate) often found in patients with AF. Although the atria continue to fibrillate with this strategy, it is nonetheless thought to be an effective treatment as it improves symptoms and reduces the risk of associated morbidity. However, the persistence of the arrhythmia continues the risk of stroke and thromboembolic events occurring. This risk is reduced by administering antithrombotic drugs (see section 7.2).

Rhythm control involves the use of electrical or pharmacological cardioversion or electro-physiological/surgical interventions to convert the arrhythmia associated with AF to normal sinus rhythm. Patients who have been successfully cardioverted are generally administered antiarrhythmic drugs for the long term to help prevent the recurrence of AF. The rhythm-control strategies also require the appropriate administration of antithrombotic therapy to reduce the risk of stroke and thromboembolic events occurring (see section 6.2).

There remain uncertainties about the most appropriate initial treatment strategy for individual patients. This section addresses which strategy is most suitable for which patient groups.

6.1.1 Methodological introduction

Five randomised controlled trials[118–122] were included in this evidence report, along with one pre-defined substudy[123] of one of the original trials. Each study compared rate-control strategies to rhythm-control strategies and involved the use of various drug therapies within each strategy.

In all rate-control treatment groups, concomitant antithrombotic therapy was administered, whereas in rhythm-control treatment groups it was administered to patients only when it was considered appropriate by the treating physician.

The follow-up periods and number of participants varied widely between the studies and only two studies[118,119] included participants who had undergone at least one previous attempt at electrical cardioversion.

None of the studies were double-blind, and in some the participants were able to swap between the different treatment groups. For example, upon multiple failed attempts at cardioversion, participants were treated according to rate-control protocols. An intention-to-treat analysis was employed in those studies where swapping was allowed.

One meta-analysis was also included.[124] Because the meta-analysis only considered the outcomes of mortality and ischaemic stroke, the results of the four primary studies will be reported for other outcomes.

Two studies[125,126] compared the cost effectiveness of the two strategies. One study[125] estimated the incremental cost per life-year gained in rhythm control versus rate control. The other study[126] estimated the cost per avoided endpoint (cardiovascular morbidity or mortality).

6.1.2 Evidence statements

For those older than 65 or those with coronary artery disease, a significant difference has been found in favour of rate control in terms of all-cause mortality.[121] (1+)

For those with heart failure (congested heart failure (CHF) or left ventricular ejection fraction (LVEF) <50%), the adoption of a rhythm-control strategy is associated with a lower incidence of all-cause mortality[121] (1+). Another study[123] reported that the overall incidence of adverse cardiovascular events in those with predominantly mild heart failure (NYHA II) was comparable between rate control and rhythm control. (1+)

Overall, a non-significant difference has been found in terms of all-cause mortality between rate and rhythm control[124] (13.0% versus 14.6%, p=0.09). (1+)

In patients with recurrent AF, a strategy of rhythm control was associated with a higher incidence of proarrhythmic events (torsades de pointes (0.8% with rhythm control versus 0.2% with rate control; p=0.007), QT prolongation (1.9% versus 0.3%; p<0.001) and bradycardic events than a strategy of rate control.[121] (1+)

In patients with recurrent AF, a strategy of rhythm control is associated with a higher rate of adverse pulmonary events (7.3% in rhythm control, 1.7% in rate control; p<0.001), gastrointestinal events (2.7% in rhythm control, 2.1% in rate control; p<0.001) or other non-cardiac adverse events (25.4% in rhythm control, 14.0% in rate control; p<0.001) than a strategy of rate control.[121] (1+)

In patients with recurrent AF, a strategy of rhythm control is associated with a higher rate of hospital admissions than is a strategy of rate control (54% versus 26%; p<0.001,[119] 74% versus 12%; p<0.001,[122] 80% versus 73%; p<0.001).[121] (1+)

In patients with recurrent AF, no significant difference has been found in quality of life,[120] myocardial infarction[121] or development of congestive heart failure[121] between strategies of rate control and rhythm control (1+); however, two studies did record a significant improvement in the level of physical functioning in both treatment groups.[119,120] (1+)

In patients with recurrent AF, no significant difference has been found in 5-year cumulative rates of thromboembolic or haemorrhagic events between strategies of rate control and rhythm control.[121] (1+)

The rate-control strategy cost US$5,077 less per person than the rhythm-control strategy (US$20,546 versus US$25,623).[125] Using low and high cost estimates in the sensitivity analysis, rate control saved from US$2,189 to US$5,481 per person. Including the mean survival gain of 0.08 of a year in rate control using original trial data, the rate-control strategy was both less costly and more effective and therefore is preferable to rhythm control.

In a study conducted in the Netherlands the rate-control strategy cost €898 less per person than the rhythm-control strategy (€7,386 versus €8,284).[126] Based on the difference in primary endpoints (cardiovascular morbidity or mortality) in rate versus rhythm control (17.5% versus

21.2%) from original trial data, rate control saves €24,944 per endpoint avoided. The higher costs with rhythm control were attributed to ECV, hospital admissions and antiarrhythmic medication.[126]

6.1.3 From evidence to recommendations

No study found rate control to be inferior to rhythm control or vice-versa for the outcome measures of mortality[118–122] or quality of life.[120] However, one study[121] found mortality to be higher for rhythm control in those with coronary heart disease, those without heart failure and those over 65 years old. The same study did not find rhythm control to be associated with lower mortality in those with heart failure.

Rates of hospitalisation, as well as rates of adverse events, were higher among participants treated with rhythm-control treatment plans.[119,121,122] The results were generally consistent across studies and considered older participants with elevated risk of stroke,[118,121] as well as younger participants.[120,122]

It was felt that many of the stroke and thromboembolic events in the rhythm-control arm were related to the lack of appropriate use of antithrombotic therapy. Rates of anticoagulation were often not controlled between the two treatment arms in many of the studies. For example, in one study[121] anticoagulation was mandatory in the rate-control treatment arm, but in the rhythm-control arm continuous anticoagulation was encouraged but could be stopped at the physician's discretion if sinus rhythm had apparently been maintained for at least 4 (and preferably 12) consecutive weeks. Anticoagulation therapy use may have had some effect on the outcome of the study, and in a subsequent post hoc analysis,[127] the use of anticoagulation therapy was an independent predictor of survival.

Although one study[121] reported a higher incidence of adverse pulmonary events associated with rhythm control, it was not reported whether this was due to the particular choice of rhythm-control drug used rather than the strategy itself.

The health economic evidence concluded that a rate-control strategy was more cost-effective than a rhythm-control strategy. However, it was unclear whether the UK setting and outcome costs of inadequate anticoagulation would affect the results.

RECOMMENDATIONS

R11 As some patients with persistent AF will satisfy criteria for either an initial rate-control or rhythm-control strategy (for example, aged over 65 but also symptomatic):
  - the indications for each option should not be regarded as mutually exclusive and the potential advantages and disadvantages of each strategy should be explained to patients before agreeing which to adopt
  - any comorbidities that might indicate one approach rather than the other should be taken into account
  - irrespective of whether a rate-control or a rhythm-control strategy is adopted in patients with persistent AF, appropriate antithrobotic therapy should be used.   D(GPP)

R12 A rate-control strategy should be the preferred initial option in the following patients with persistent AF:

- over 65 years old   B
- with coronary artery disease   B
- with contraindications to antiarrhythmic drugs   D(GPP)
- unsuitable for cardioversion*   D(GPP)
- without congestive heart failure.   B

R13 A rhythm-control strategy should be the preferred initial option in the following patients with persistent AF:

- those who are symptomatic   D(GPP)
- younger patients   C
- those presenting for the first time with lone AF   D(GPP)
- those with AF secondary to a treated/corrected precipitant D(GPP)
- those with congestive heart failure.   C

*Patients unsuitable for cardioversion include those with:
- contraindications to anticoagulation
- structural heart disease (eg large left atrium >5.5 cm, mitral stenosis) that precludes long-term maintenance of sinus rhythm
- a long duration of AF (usually >12 months)
- a history of multiple failed attempts at cardioversion and/or relapses, even with concomitant use of antiarrhythmic drugs or non-pharmacological approaches
- an ongoing but reversible cause of atrial fibrillation (eg thyrotoxicosis).

6.2 Rhythm control for persistent AF

In persistent AF, antiarrhythmic drugs are prescribed to increase the likelihood of maintaining sinus rhythm following successful electrical or pharmacological cardioversion.

The use of antiarrhythmic drugs to maintain sinus rhythm post cardioversion is addressed in this section. In UK clinical practice, prophylactic drug treatment is not usually used in cases of a first-detected episode of AF, especially if AF is secondary to a precipitant that has since been corrected. Without antiarrhythmic drugs, the recurrence rate is high. Reversible cardiovascular and non-cardiovascular precipitants of AF are usually actively managed first. Predictors of recurrences of AF are considered elsewhere (see section 12.2).

Clinical studies have shown the efficacy of various antiarrhythmic drugs (amiodarone, propafenone, disopyramide, sotalol, flecainide, quinidine and azimilide) against no treatment, placebo or digoxin.[64,68,128] It is clear from these trials that the use of antiarrhythmic drugs does improve maintenance of sinus rhythm post cardioversion. But despite treatment, relapse to AF occurs in approximately 50% of patients by 12 months (see section 12.2). Moreover, the need for antiarrhythmic drugs has to be balanced against adverse effects and a higher mortality in some patients.[129]

UK clinical practice commonly uses Class Ic, beta-blockers or Class III antiarrhythmic drugs to maintain sinus rhythm, and this section compares their relative efficacy.

6.2.1 Methodological introduction

The literature search and evidence appraisal processes for this question resulted in 12 studies being included in this evidence report.

Studies were considered for inclusion if the efficacy of antiarrhythmic drugs was measured in a study population or subpopulation with a history of AF requiring electrical or chemical cardioversion, and an indication for long-term antiarrhythmic therapy for the maintenance of sinus rhythm.

Studies that consider the use of antiarrhythmic therapy specifically for reducing the frequency of recurrent episodes of AF in those patients with a history of paroxysmal AF are considered elsewhere (see section 8.1).

All but two[111,130] of the studies included in this report were RCTs.

No studies compared the efficacy of amiodarone, flecainide or propafenone with a beta-blocker such as metoprolol. However, five studies[89,111,131–133] compared amiodarone with the Class III beta-blocker sotalol, and three studies[134–136] compared propafenone with sotalol. Two studies[130,137] compared a Class Ic agent (flecainide or propafenone) with amiodarone. One study[112] compared amiodarone with either sotalol or propafenone, and one study[138] compared sotalol with the beta-blocker bisoprolol.

All studies except one[138] explicitly excluded patients with severe heart failure. Most also excluded those with moderate heart failure (typically defined as an NYHA grade greater than II).

Most of the studies were not powered to detect clinically significant differences in drug side effects, and many reported the composite endpoint of either recurrence of AF or occurrence of a drug-related side effect or drug withdrawal.

6.2.2 Evidence statements

▷ Sotalol versus propafenone

Two studies[134,135] found no difference in the proportion of patients with AF maintaining sinus rhythm at 12 months between sotalol and propafenone (1+). One study[135] also found a similar result when only those subgroups with a history of paroxysmal or persistent AF were considered. (1+)

One study[136] found propafenone resulted in a lower incidence of side effects or AF recurrence than sotalol (52% versus 81%; p<0.001). (1+)

▷ Sotalol versus amiodarone

Three studies[89,131,132] found amiodarone to be significantly associated with an increased likelihood of remaining in sinus rhythm compared with sotalol at 12[89,131,132] and 24[132] months following cardioversion (1++). Similar results were found for the likelihood of remaining in sinus rhythm without side effects[111,132] and the monthly incidence of AF recurrence or side effects.[133] (1+)

One study[89] also found amiodarone to be associated with an increased likelihood of remaining in sinus rhythm compared with sotalol regardless of the duration of AF and whether or not the AF was associated with symptoms (1++). However, the study found no significant difference between the two drugs in those patients with ischaemic heart disease. (1++)

▷ Sotalol versus beta-blockers

One study[138] found no difference in the percentage of patients with recurrent AF during a mean follow-up period of approximately 8 months between 5 mg/day bisoprolol and 160 mg/day sotalol (42% versus 41%) (1+). There were two cases of proarrhythmia and two cases of bradycardia in the sotalol group and two cases of bradycardia in the bisoprolol group.

▷ Flecainide versus amiodarone

One study[130] of patients with recurrent AF found no significant difference in the efficacy of flecainide and amiodarone over a period of 3 months in terms of the rate of recurrent AF (38% versus 32%). (2++)

▷ Propafenone versus amiodarone

One study[112] comparing either propafenone or sotalol with amiodarone found amiodarone to be associated with a higher proportion of patients remaining in sinus rhythm after an average follow-up period of 468 days (39% versus 69%; p<0.001) (1+). Sotalol and propafenone were similar in terms of efficacy. Amiodarone was also associated with a lower incidence of drug-related side effects requiring discontinuation compared with sotalol/propafenone (46% versus 34%; p=0.01), although the incidence of drug discontinuation between the propafenone and sotalol patients was not reported separately. (1+)

One study[137] found no significant difference between propafenone and amiodarone in terms of the percentage of patients maintaining sinus rhythm over 24 months (52% versus 59%; p=0.058) (1+). When the composite outcome of remaining in sinus rhythm without side effects was considered, the two drugs were similar (51% versus 42%; p=0.44). (1+)

6.2.3 From evidence to recommendations

An escalating approach to drug therapy could be recommended based on associated comorbidity and the need for increasingly effective antiarrhythmic drugs. For example, a beta-blocker or sotalol could be prescribed in the first instance, and where this was not tolerated, or was ineffective, other drugs could be administered.

This escalation of drug use is not totally in keeping with the evidence on efficacy, which is in favour of amiodarone, but also incorporates concerns regarding the adverse effects. In the case of amiodarone, such adverse effects may become apparent only after long-term use and include pulmonary, hepatic, ophthalmic and thyroid toxicity.

RECOMMENDATIONS

R14   An antiarrhythmic drug is not required to maintain sinus rhythm in patients with persistent AF in whom a precipitant (such as chest infection or fever) has been corrected and cardioversion has been performed successfully, providing there are no risk factors for recurrence.   D(GPP)

R15   In patients with persistent AF who require antiarrhythmic drugs to maintain sinus rhythm and who have structural heart disease*:

- a standard beta-blocker should be the initial treatment option   D(GPP)
- where a standard beta-blocker is ineffective, contraindicated or not tolerated amiodarone should be used.   A

R16   In patients with persistent AF who require antiarrhythmic drugs to maintain sinus rhythm and who do not have structural heart disease*:

- a standard beta-blocker should be the initial treatment option   D(GPP)
- where a standard beta-blocker is ineffective, contraindicated or not tolerated
    - a Class Ic agent or   C
    - sotalol**   D(GPP)

should be given

- where other drug classes are ineffective, contraindicated or not tolerated amiodarone should be administered.   B

*Coronary artery disease or left ventricular dysfunction.
**Progressively titrated from 80 mg twice daily up to 240 mg twice daily.

6.3 Antithrombotic therapy for persistent AF

Patients with persistent AF may be treated with either a rate-control or rhythm-control treatment strategy. Where a rhythm-control treatment strategy is chosen, there is the need for appropriate use of antithrombotic therapy to prevent acute stroke or other thromboembolic events occurring during or shortly after cardioversion. Where a rate-control strategy is chosen, patients should be treated as outlined for permanent AF (see Chapter 7).

It is known that the presence of AF increases the risk of thromboembolic stroke,[13] but it is less clear whether this risk can be reduced by cardioversion (ECV or PCV) to normal sinus rhythm, assuming sinus rhythm is maintained and antithrombotic therapy is continued. The rate-versus rhythm-control trials have not resolved this issue as many of the patients relapsed into AF and had been administered inadequate thromboprophylaxis (see section 6.1).

Appropriate thromboprophylactic measures are essential in patients considered for cardioversion since it has been shown that cardioversion of AF of more than 48 hours duration increases the short-term (peri-cardioversion) risk of stroke and thromboembolism.[139,140] Data from the rate-control versus rhythm-control trials suggest that consideration should be given to long-term anticoagulation in patients at high risk of stroke and/or AF recurrence in view of the frequent asymptomatic recurrences of the arrhythmia leading to thromboembolism in the presence of risk factors.[65]

In the past, there have been no prospective randomised placebo-controlled trials testing the efficacy of anticoagulation (versus placebo) in the prevention of peri-cardioversion thromboembolism, but several retrospective studies and/or case series have suggested benefit from the use of therapeutic warfarin in this setting. Cardioversion of atrial flutter presents similar risks and requires similar anticoagulation.

The administration of antithrombotic therapy peri-cardioversion applies to both electrical and pharmacological cardioversion strategies.

Apart from the periods leading up to and following cardioversion, there is no evidence to suggest that the choice of antithrombotic therapy should be any different from that recommended for patients with permanent AF (see section 7.2).

6.3.1 Methodological introduction

The results of a meta-analysis of 25 primary studies[141] and three primary studies[142–144] are included in this report. Only one[144] of the primary studies was a RCT.

The meta-analysis included in this report[141] pooled the results of multiple primary studies comparing the effectiveness of anticoagulation or the effectiveness of TOE screening for the prevention of acute embolic events (ischaemic stroke or transient ischaemic attack or systemic embolism) post cardioversion.

None of the studies examined rates of thromboembolism in emergency versus elective cardioversion, and in particular whether acute anticoagulation with heparinoids is an effective means of stroke prevention in comparison to oral anticoagulation.

No studies compared the effectiveness of any form of anticoagulation post cardioversion against placebo or the effectiveness of antiplatelet agents against either anticoagulation or placebo.

6.3.2 Evidence statements

Based on the results of two primary studies[142,143] and one meta-analysis,[141] anticoagulation prior to cardioversion has been found to be associated with a reduced rate of thromboembolic complications post cardioversion when compared with no anticoagulation. (2++)

Anticoagulation reaching an international normalised ratio (INR) greater than 2.0 at the time of cardioversion has been found to be associated with a significantly lower rate of thromboembolic complications 4 weeks post cardioversion when compared with lower values (including those receiving no anticoagulation).[142,143] (2+)

Anticoagulation prior to cardioversion has been found to be associated with a reduced rate of acute thromboembolic complications post cardioversion when compared with TOE screening for the presence of thrombi prior to cardioversion and the exclusion of screen-positive patients.[141] (2++)

Anticoagulation with enoxaparin throughout the peri-cardioversion period is as effective as unfractionated heparin peri-cardioversion followed by oral anticoagulation with a coumarin derivative post cardioversion.[144] (1+)

6.3.3   From evidence to recommendations

Anticoagulation administered to a target INR of 2.5 (with a range of 2.0 to 3.0) prior to cardioversion is effective in reducing the frequency of acute thromboembolic complications post cardioversion. In studies involving anticoagulation to resolve any intracardiac thombi, a duration of 3 to 4 weeks prior to cardioversion has often been specified.[114,145] It was therefore considered necessary for anticoagulation to be therapeutic (within the INR range 2.0 to 3.0) for a minimum of 3 weeks prior to cardioversion for resolution or endothelisation of any pre-existing thrombus. In practice this may be verified as three consecutive weekly INR measurements within the therapeutic range.

Anticoagulation is more effective than screening patients for thrombi using TOE alone as a means of reducing the frequency of thromboembolic complications of cardioversion.[141]

Based on a period of 4 weeks for the return of atrial contractile function post cardioversion, it was considered that anticoagulation should remain at therapeutic levels throughout this time. Even in patients with a successful cardioversion, evidence from the AFFIRM study[121,127] suggests that longer-term anticoagulation may be necessary in the presence of stroke and thromboembolism risk factors (see section 11.6) or risk factors for AF recurrence (see section 12.2). The evidence from AFFIRM showed that, although sinus rhythm is associated with reduced mortality, patients enrolled in the rhythm-control treatment strategy had a similar incidence of stroke to those in the rate-control treatment strategy.

It is noteworthy that many of the risk factors for thromboembolism in AF are similar to those for AF recurrence.

RECOMMENDATIONS

R17   Before cardioversion, patients should be maintained on therapeutic anticoagulation with warfarin (INR 2.5, range 2.0 to 3.0) for a minimum of 3 weeks.   C

R18   Following successful cardioversion, patients should remain on therapeutic anticoagulation with warfarin (INR 2.5, range 2.0 to 3.0) for a minimum of 4 weeks.   D(GPP)

R19   In patients with persistent AF where cardioversion cannot be postponed for 3 weeks:
   • heparin should be given and the cardioversion performed, and   D
   • warfarin should then be given for a minimum of 4 weeks post cardioversion.   D(GPP)

R20   Anticoagulation should be continued for the long term in patients with AF who have undergone cardioversion where there is a high risk of AF recurrence* or where it is recommended by the stroke risk stratification algorithm (Figure 11.1).   D(GPP)

R21   In patients with AF of confirmed duration of less than 48 hours undergoing cardioversion, anticoagulation following successful restoration of sinus rhythm is not required.   D(GPP)

R22   Patients with atrial flutter should be given antithrombotic therapy in the same manner as those with AF.   D(GPP)

*Factors indicating a high risk of AF recurrence include:
   • a history of failed attempts at cardioversion
   • structural heart disease (mitral valve disease, left ventricular dysfunction or an enlarged left atrium)
   • a prolonged history of AF (greater than 12 months)
   • previous recurrences of AF.

6.4   Rhythm-control treatment algorithm for persistent AF

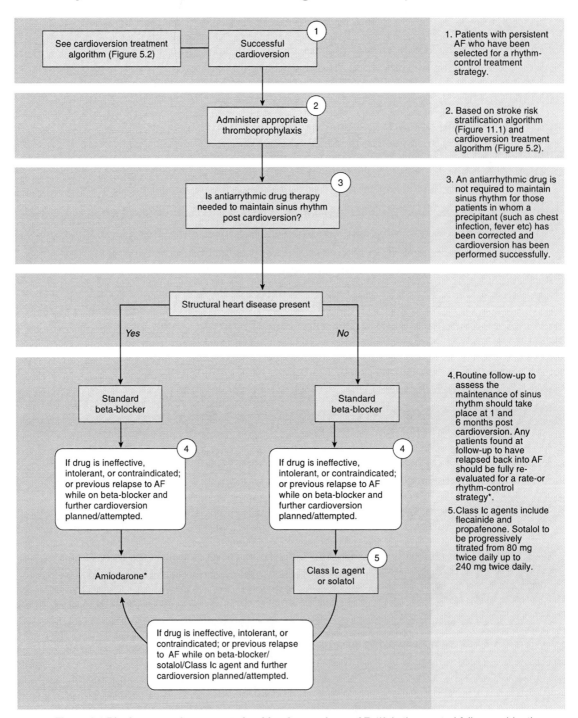

Figure 6.1 Rhythm-control treatment algorithm for persistent AF. *If rhythm control fails, consider the patient for rate-control strategy or specialist referral in those with lone AF or ECG evidence of underlying electrophysiological disorder (eg Wolff–Parkinson–White syndrome).

7 Treatment for permanent AF

7.1 Rate control for permanent AF

The aims of heart rate control are to minimise symptoms associated with excessive heart rates and prevent tachycardia-associated cardiomyopathy.[146] A recent consensus[147] statement has suggested a target resting heart rate of less than 90 bpm and less than 180 bpm during exercise in patients with AF.

Historically, cardiac glycosides such as digoxin have been used but have limited efficacy in a hyperadrenergic state such as thyrotoxicosis, fever, acute volume loss, postoperative state and during exertion.[148] In clinical practice, digoxin monotherapy may only be adequate for the older, sedentary patient.[149] Other agents for rate control include beta-blockers and the rate-limiting non-dihydropyridine calcium-channel blockers ('calcium antagonists') such as diltiazem and verapamil. These are used for rate control, both at rest and during exercise, and are perceived to be more effective than digoxin in the critically ill.[65,150] Diltiazem is regarded as preferable to verapamil, in view of the latter's negative inotropic effect and potential drug interaction with digoxin. Beta-blockers and calcium antagonists may also worsen acute heart failure.

One short acting intravenous beta-blocker, esmolol, is useful when oral drugs cannot be given or if there is uncertainty over tolerance of the beta-blocker.

Rate control may not always be achieved with a single drug. Combination therapy, for example digoxin plus a beta-blocker or rate-limiting calcium-channel blocker is often considered for AF uncontrolled with a single agent. If these two classes of drugs are ineffective or not tolerated, amiodarone or diltiazem-beta-blocker combination therapy are third-line pharmacological options used by specialists. Alternatively, a non-pharmacological approach (mainly atrio-ventricular node ablation coupled with pacing) can be considered, but is beyond the scope of this review.

7.1.1 Methodological introduction

This section considered the efficacy of:
* beta-blockers,
* digoxin and
* calcium antagonists.

Of the 12 studies that were included, all but one[151] were either randomised or serial crossover trials. Consequently, the total number of participants was relatively low.

For the comparison of calcium antagonists and beta-blockers, three studies were found, one of which[152] used the beta-blocker betaxolol, which is not available orally in the UK. In this and a second study,[153] the patients were also receiving digoxin, which may have confounded the results.

There is consistency in the results between different drugs within the same class for both the comparison of calcium antagonists versus digoxin and beta-blockers versus digoxin.

7.1.2   Evidence statements

▷ Calcium antagonists versus digoxin

Seven studies[154–160] found no difference in average heart rate between calcium antagonists verapamil or diltiazem and digoxin either at rest or during periods of normal daily activity (1++). However, seven studies[153,155–160] found calcium antagonists resulted in a lower heart rate during exercise, compared with digoxin. (1++)

▷ Beta-blockers versus digoxin

Three studies[151,154,161] found no difference in average heart rate between digoxin and beta-blockers while at rest or during periods of normal daily activity (1++). However, the beta-blockers atenolol[154] and labetalol[161] controlled heart rate during exercise more effectively than digoxin did (1++). One additional study[153] found that atenolol significantly reduced average heart rate in comparison to digoxin both at rest and after exercise. (1+)

▷ Beta-blockers versus calcium antagonists

One crossover study[154] found no difference between the calcium antagonist diltiazem and the beta-blocker atenolol in terms of either the mean heart rate over 24 hours or during exercise (1+). A second crossover study[153] found no difference in the mean heart rate at rest or post-exercise between the calcium antagonist verapamil and atenolol (1+). However, a third study[152] found the beta-blocker betaxolol to be more effective than diltiazem both over 24 hours and during exercise. (1+)

▷ Beta-blockers with digoxin versus beta-blockers

One crossover study[154] found the beta-blocker atenolol used in combination with digoxin to be associated with a lower heart rate over 24 hours than atenolol alone (1+). In another study[161] using the beta-blocker labetalol the reported differences were not statistically significant (1++). Neither study found any statistically significant differences in heart rate during periods of exercise. (1++)

▷ Calcium antagonists with digoxin versus calcium antagonists

Four crossover studies[154,156,159,162] found the calcium antagonists diltiazem or verapamil used in combination with digoxin to be more effective in controlling heart rate over 24 hours, as well as during periods of exercise, than either diltiazem or verapamil alone. (1++)

7.1.3   From evidence to recommendations

When used as monotherapies, both calcium antagonists and beta-blockers were more effective than digoxin in controlling heart rate at high levels of physical exertion, but there was no difference during normal daily activities. Based on the results of two studies there was no significant difference in terms of the effectiveness of heart rate control between calcium antagonists and beta-blockers.[152,154]

During rest the combination of beta-blockers with digoxin was more effective than beta-blockers alone for the control of heart rate.[154,161] The combination of calcium antagonists with digoxin was more effective than calcium antagonists alone for the control of heart rate both during normal activities and rest, as well as during exercise.[154,156,159]

None of the studies were sufficiently large to make comparisons in terms of side effects. In particular, no study reported any intolerance to beta-blockers.

RECOMMENDATIONS

R23   In patients with permanent AF, who need treatment for rate control:

- beta-blockers or rate-limiting calcium antagonists should be the preferred initial monotherapy in all patients   **A**
- digoxin should only be considered as monotherapy in predominately sedentary patients.   **D(GPP)**

R24   In patients with permanent AF where monotherapy is inadequate:

- to control the heart rate only during normal activities, beta-blockers or rate-limiting calcium antagonists should be given with digoxin   **B**
- to control the heart rate during both normal activities and exercise, rate-limiting calcium antagonists should be given with digoxin.   **B**

7.2   Antithrombotic therapy for permanent AF

The aim of antithrombotic therapy in patients with permanent AF is to prevent ischaemic stroke and other thromboembolic events. This section examines which type of antithrombotic therapy (anticoagulation, antiplatelet drugs or no treatment) has been shown to be effective in treating patients with permanent AF.

The high risk of ischaemic stroke and other thromboembolic events in AF has long been recognised. In particular, AF patients with valvular heart disease have an elevated risk of stroke and other thromboembolic events. Specifically, the presence of mitral valve stenosis has been shown to be a substantial risk for stroke and thromboembolism, with these events occurring in 9 to 20% of patients, of whom up to 75% have cerebral emboli.[163,164] A person with mitral stenosis in sinus rhythm who develops AF increases their risk of thromboembolism by three to seven times.[164,165] The risk of systemic emboli in rheumatic mitral disease is much greater in both the elderly and those with poor cardiac function, but correlates poorly with mitral valve calcification, mitral valve area, or left atrial size.

Percutaneous balloon mitral commissurotomy decreases the risk of systemic embolism, but mitral valvuloplasty does not appear to. Successful mitral valvuloplasty does not therefore eliminate the need for continued anticoagulation.[164] Because of the risk of stroke and thromboembolism, it has been considered unethical to conduct placebo-controlled trials of antithrombotic therapy in patients with mitral valve disease.

Similarly, the presence of AF without any valve disease (non-valvular AF) increases the risk of stroke and thromboembolism five-fold.[13] Silent cerebral infarction is also a common problem[166] and there is a distinct clustering of stroke events at the time of onset of AF as well.[167] In contrast to valvular AF, however, in the past two decades many large randomised trials have examined the value of antithrombotic therapy in non-valvular AF.[168]

Because of the increasingly elderly population, AF is likely to become more common, and the issues associated with thromboprophylaxis will become an even greater public health problem. Despite the higher risk associated with stroke in the elderly, as well as the greatest benefit of anticoagulation, the elderly are the group of patients where there is suboptimal use of thromboprophylaxis for AF. This is thought to be because of the perceived increased risk associated with comorbidity, interactions with concomitant drug therapies and bleeding in these patients.[169] Suboptimal use of thromboprophylaxis may also be due to patient factors, where some patients choose the option of 'informed dissent' and decline an effective treatment option.[170]

The purpose of this section is to review the evidence on antithrombotic therapies (oral anti-coagulation and/or antiplatelet therapy) as a means of preventing stroke and thromboembolism in patients with permanent AF.

7.2.1 Methodological introduction

The results of eight meta-analyses, four RCTs and two unrandomised controlled trials of oral anticoagulation using vitamin K antagonists such as warfarin, and antiplatelet therapy in patients with AF were included. Results relating to the antiplatelet agent triflusal were included but no recommendations were made on this drug as it is not currently licensed for use in the UK.

Most of the trials were large randomised trials, consisting almost entirely of patients with permanent non-valvular AF.

7.2.2 Evidence statements

▷ Adjusted-dose warfarin versus placebo

Two studies,[171,172] found that compared with placebo, adjusted-dose warfarin was associated with a reduction in ischaemic stroke: (1+)
- ARR = 3.1% (62% RRR)[171]
- OR = 0.34 (95% CI 0.25 to 0.46).[172]

However, in one study adjusted-dose warfarin was found to be associated with an increased risk of major haemorrhage (OR 2.35, 95% CI 1.30 to 4.24)[172] (1+). The same study[172] also found no significant difference in terms of overall mortality (OR 0.74, 95% CI 0.53 to 1.04). (1+)

▷ Adjusted-dose warfarin versus control treatment (aspirin or placebo)

One study[173] found adjusted-dose warfarin (compared with aspirin or placebo controls) to be associated with a significant reduction in the incidence of ischaemic stroke as well as the composite outcomes of haemorrhagic or ischaemic stroke, and vascular events (myocardial infarction, stroke, haemorrhage, vascular death) (1+). The same study[173] also found no significant effect for the incidence of myocardial infarction, systemic embolism or intracranial haemorrhage (ICH). (1+)

▷ Adjusted-dose warfarin versus antiplatelet therapy (aspirin or indobufen)

Two meta-analyses[171,174] found adjusted-dose warfarin (compared with antiplatelet therapy with aspirin or indobufen) to be significantly associated with an absolute risk reduction of ischaemic stroke: (1+)

- ARR = 0.8% (36% RRR), $p<0.05$[171]
- ARR = 2.3% (2.0% versus 4.3%; $p<0.001$).[174]

One meta-analysis[174] found that when the composite outcome of either ischaemic stroke or ICH was considered, it resulted in an absolute risk reduction of 2.1% (2.4% versus 4.5%; $p<0.001$). (1+)

In one meta-analyses[174] adjusted-dose warfarin was found to be associated with an increase in incidence of major haemorrhage (increased absolute risk of 0.9% (2.2% versus 1.3%; $p<0.05$)), however, in a second meta-analysis no significant difference was found.[175] (1+)

One study[175] found adjusted-dose warfarin (compared with antiplatelet therapy with aspirin or indobufen) to be associated with a reduced incidence of non-fatal stroke, although no significant difference has been found for fatal stroke, nor overall mortality (1+). In another study,[176] adjusted-dose warfarin was found to be associated with a reduced incidence of severe ischaemic stroke in those where an ischaemic stroke occurs. (2+)

▷ Adjusted-dose warfarin versus fixed, low-dose warfarin

One meta-analysis[172] found adjusted-dose warfarin to be associated with a reduced risk of stroke (OR 0.38, 95% CI 0.24 to 0.60) compared with fixed, low-dose warfarin. In a second study[177] only the composite outcome of all thrombotic events was found to be significant (RR 0.50, 95% CI 0.25 to 0.97). (1+)

No significant difference has been found in the incidence of overall mortality,[172] vascular or haemorrhagic death[177] or major haemorrhage[172] between fixed, low-dose warfarin and adjusted-dose warfarin. (1+)

▷ Adjusted-dose warfarin versus fixed, low-dose warfarin with aspirin

One meta-analysis[172] found adjusted-dose warfarin (compared with fixed, low-dose warfarin) significantly reduced the incidence of stroke (OR 0.38, 95% CI 0.24 to 0.60). However a larger meta-analysis[177] found no significant difference (1+). No significant difference has been found in terms of overall mortality,[172] vascular or haemorrhagic death[177] or major haemorrhage[172] between fixed, low-dose warfarin with aspirin and adjusted-dose warfarin (1+)

One study[176] found that at an INR greater than or equal to 2.0, adjusted-dose warfarin was associated with a reduced incidence of severe ischaemic stroke in those where an ischaemic stroke occurs compared with when the INR is less than 2.0. (2+)

▷ Antiplatelet therapy with aspirin or dipyridamole and placebo

Based on the results of two studies,[172,178] no significant difference has been found between antiplatelet therapy with aspirin or dipyridamole and placebo in terms of:

- overall mortality[172] (1+)
- vascular death[178] (1+)
- myocardial infarction[178] (1+)
- systemic embolism[178] (1+)
- vascular event[178] (1+)
- major haemorrhage.[172,178] (1+)

One meta-analysis[171] found antiplatelet therapy to be associated with an absolute risk reduction for stroke of 1.9% (24% relative risk reduction), however, in two smaller meta-analyses[172,178] no significant differences were found. (1+)

▷ Triflusal with acenocoumarol versus acenocoumarol monotherapy

One study[179] which compared triflusal (600 mg per day) in combination with acenocoumarol (INR of 1.25 to 2.00) with acenocoumarol monotherapy (INR of 2.0 to 3.0) found that the composite outcome of overall (haemorrhagic and ischaemic) stroke incidence, vascular death or systemic embolism was lower in the combination therapy group than in the acenocoumarol monotherapy group (0.92% per year versus 2.70% per year; p<0.05) (1+). A similar association was found when the number of severe bleeding events was added to the overall incidence of stroke or systemic embolism (1.48% per year versus 3.78% per year; p<0.05) (1+). No statistically significant difference was reported in the incidence of severe bleeding events. (1+)

7.2.3   From evidence to recommendations

The studies included wide variations in the dose of aspirin (75 mg to 325 mg per day). Similarly, the studies differed in the degree of anticoagulation, with earlier studies using a higher level of anticoagulation (INR range of 2.0 to 4.5) than more recent studies.

Oral anticoagulation with vitamin K antagonists (such as warfarin) was the most effective thromboprophylactic treatment in the prevention of cardioembolic stroke. A target INR of 2.5 (range 2 to 3) should be maintained for the majority of patients.[176] However, anticoagulation is associated with an increased rate of haemorrhagic stroke and other bleeding events.[172] Nonetheless, it remains effective for the prevention of stroke overall.[174,175] No association between anticoagulation and mortality has been found for either vascular-related deaths[173] or all forms of death.[172]

The true efficacy of warfarin prophylaxis may have been underestimated as most strokes in patients randomised to warfarin occurred when the patients were not taking warfarin or when they were significantly under-anticoagulated. Further underestimates may have risen from the inconvenience of dosing adjustments and the need for regular blood tests to monitor INR levels, dietary restrictions, the risk of minor and major bleeding, and under-appreciation or lack of knowledge of the risk of stroke, or they may not adhere strictly to the treatment regimen, thereby placing themselves at greater risk for stroke or a major bleed.[169,180]

The dose of aspirin for AF thromboprophylaxis is subject to controversy. The relative stroke risk reduction of aspirin in AF patients is approximately 22%.[171] This is similar to that seen in a general population and the reduction of vascular events (22%) for antiplatelet therapy versus control in 'high risk' patients with vascular disease.[181] Moreover, in the latter cases no differences have been reported in aspirin doses between 75 to 325 mg.[181] However, higher aspirin doses may be associated with more adverse effects.

AF commonly co-exists with vascular disease, and the benefits of aspirin in AF may simply relate to the effect on vascular disease, rather than on thrombogenesis in AF *per se*. This is supported by the thrombi associated with AF being fibrin rich ('red clot') and more related to coagulation abnormalities.

In trials specifically of AF populations comparing aspirin with placebo, the one trial[182] that tested aspirin 75 mg/day did not show a significant benefit for the prevention of stroke in patients with permanent AF. Similarly, in another trial[183] aspirin (most at 325 mg per day) was given in a non-randomised manner, and no significant benefit was seen. However, in another trial[184] using aspirin 325 mg/day, aspirin was reported to result in a significant 42% reduction in stroke, but was best for those aged under 75 years and did not prevent severe strokes or recurrent strokes.

Because aspirin 325 mg tablets are unavailable in the UK, and in view of the controversy over trial evidence in relation to the pathophysiological data, it was considered reasonable to recommend the use of aspirin at a dose of 75 to 300 mg/day as thromboprophylaxis.

It was noted that the addition of aspirin to oral anticoagulation (warfarin or fluindione) produced no extra benefit for stroke prevention but may increase bleeding risk. It was therefore felt that to prevent strokes in patients with AF, aspirin should not be given as adjunctive therapy to warfarin although there may be other reasons for co-prescribing aspirin. For example, aspirin 75 mg a day is commonly prescribed for vascular disease (eg carotid, coronary or peripheral artery disease), and if AF is also present, warfarin – if indicated for stroke prevention – is also commonly given. It is a matter for clinical judgement on the appropriateness, duration and safety (eg risk of bleeding) of the concomitant administration of warfarin with aspirin. It was noted that another antiplatelet agent (trifusal, not available in the UK) was of benefit when administered together with the oral anticoagulant acenocoumarol.

It was stressed that the risk of stroke and thromboembolism in AF patients is not homogeneous, and risk stratification is essential (see section 11.6).

RECOMMENDATIONS

R25   In patients with permanent AF a risk–benefit assessment should be performed and discussed with the patient to inform the decision whether or not to give antithrombotic therapy.   D(GPP)

R26   In patients with permanent AF where antithrombotic therapy is given to prevent strokes and/or thromboembolism (see section 11.6):
   - adjusted-dose warfarin should be given as the most effective treatment   A
   - adjusted-dose warfarin should reach a target INR of 2.5 (range 2.0 to 3.0)   A
   - where warfarin is not appropriate, aspirin should be given at 75 to 300 mg/day   B
   - where warfarin is appropriate, aspirin should not be co-administered with warfarin purely as thromboprophylaxis, as it provides no additional benefit.   B

7.3   Rate-control treatment algorithm for permanent AF

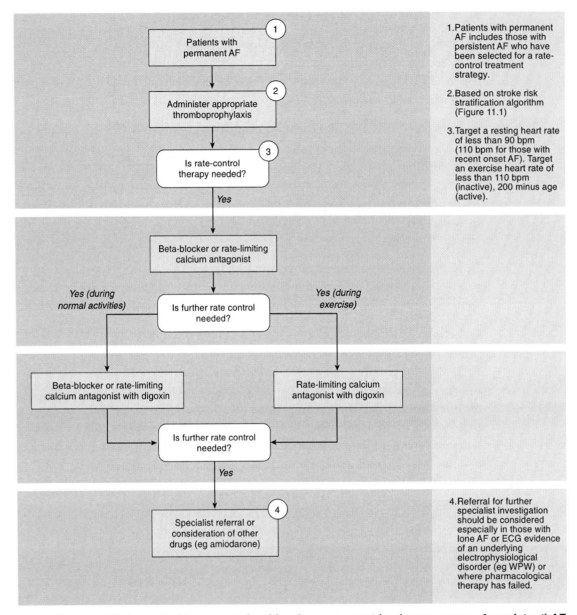

Figure 7.1 Rate-control treatment algorithm for permanent (and some cases of persistent) AF

8 Treatment for paroxysmal AF

8.1 Rhythm control for paroxysmal AF

The three main aims of treatment for paroxysmal AF are:

(i) to suppress paroxysms of AF and maintain long-term sinus rhythm

(ii) to control heart rate during paroxysms of AF if they occur

(iii) to prevent the complications associated with paroxysmal AF, ie stroke- and tachycardia-induced cardiomyopathy.[185]

This section of the guideline essentially deals with the first aim.

Many patients with paroxysmal AF can be highly symptomatic.[31] Paroxysms of AF that are persistent (that is, lasting more than 7 days) can be considered for cardioversion to sinus rhythm (see Chapter 5).

However, the abolition of symptoms of paroxysmal AF does not necessarily mean abolition of the AF *per se*, as heart rate slowing may abolish symptoms but allow asymptomatic episodes to continue.[186] In patients with symptomatic recurrences, it may be appropriate to document the frequency of arrhythmia by Holter monitoring or event recording (see section 4.4 above). If symptoms are abolished by therapy, repeat monitoring to ascertain whether asymptomatic episodes of AF are present is occasionally performed.

If attacks of paroxysmal AF are frequent, in current clinical practice chronic prophylaxis is usually used with drugs to reduce the frequency of paroxysms after removal of precipitating factors such as caffeine, alcohol, stress, and adequate treatment of underlying diseases such as myocardial ischaemia, thyrotoxicosis and heart failure.[185] If episodes of paroxysmal AF are infrequent, a pill-in-the-pocket approach can be considered (see section 8.2).

In the long term, few patients achieve complete suppression of paroxysms of AF. In clinical practice, clinicians commonly use beta-blockers or low-dose sotalol as first-line drugs, and if the patient is still getting symptomatic paroxysms, Class Ic and III drugs are used, depending on associated comorbidity and structural heart disease.

In UK clinical practice, the drugs commonly used for paroxysmal AF are beta-blockers, Class Ic agents (flecainide, propafenone) and Class III agents (sotalol, amiodarone). This section addresses the comparative efficacy of these agents.

8.1.1 Methodological introduction

Studies were considered for inclusion in this report if results were reported for a population or subpopulation with paroxysmal AF. Studies were excluded if the treatment drugs were not prescribed as regular medication for paroxysmal AF.

Nine studies were appraised, two[187,188] were entirely comprised of paroxysmal AF patients, although the follow-up times were relatively short (12 months or less) compared with other studies in a general AF population. The remaining studies were undertaken in general AF populations and either reported the results for those with paroxysmal AF separately, or reported no significant interaction between AF type and drug efficacy, hence allowing extrapolation of the results to those with paroxysmal AF only.

All of the studies were either single-blinded or double-blinded RCTs with two active treatment arms. Studies that made comparisons with placebo or digoxin were not considered. All of the studies excluded patients with moderate-to-severe heart failure (typically defined as an NYHA grade greater than II).

One study based in Canada compared the costs of amiodarone treatment with propafenone/sotalol treatment.[189] The cost analysis was based on 1-year follow-up data of 392 patients randomised to low-dose amiodarone (200 mg/day) or alternative first-line therapy (sotalol or propafenone) in a multicentre open label trial.[112]

8.1.2 Evidence statements

▷ Propafenone versus sotalol

One study[187] found no significant difference in the proportion of patients experiencing a reduction in recurrent AF episodes between propafenone and sotalol (80 to 160 mg bid) over a minimum of 3 months. (1++)

One study[136] showed a significant difference in terms of the proportion of patients maintaining sinus rhythm between propafenone and sotalol (up to 480 mg/day) in favour of propafenone after 25 months of administration (1+). However, over shorter periods two other studies[134,135] found no significant difference. (1++)

One study[187] involving both persistent and paroxysmal AF participants found no significant difference in the rates of either intolerable or tolerable side effects between sotalol (80 to 160 mg bid) and propafenone. (1++)

▷ Amiodarone versus sotalol

Two studies involving subgroups of patients with paroxysmal AF[132,133] found amiodarone to be significantly associated with a lower rate of AF recurrence[133] and a higher prevalence of sinus rhythm[132] at 12 months and at 24 months compared to sotalol (160 to 480 mg/day[132] or 160 to 320 mg/day[133]). (1+)

▷ Beta-blockers versus sotalol

One small, open-label crossover study[188] found no significant difference between atenolol and sotalol (80 mg bid) in the frequency of recurrent episodes of AF or the average duration of recurrent episodes. (1+)

▷ Propafenone versus amiodarone

One study,[112] in a population of both persistent and paroxysmal AF patients, found amiodarone to be significantly associated with a higher prevalence of sinus rhythm at a mean follow-up of approximately 15.6 months compared with propafenone or sotalol (69% versus 39%, respectively; p<0.001) (1+). The same study also reported comparable efficacy between propafenone and sotalol, as well as comparable outcomes in each arm of the study for paroxysmal and persistent AF patients (1+). In another study[137] involving a subgroup of 92 patients with paroxysmal AF, 40% of those treated with amiodarone had a recurrence of AF at 24 months, compared with 83% of those treated with propafenone (p=0.19) (1+). When the composite endpoint of either AF recurrence or occurrence of side effects was considered, the figures were 58% versus 53%, respectively (p=0.51). (1+)

One study[189] found that the average cost per patient for AF-related procedures and hospitalisations was significantly lower in the amiodarone group than the sotalol/propafenone group (US$532 versus US$898, p=0.03). This cost advantage increased when the costs of hospitalisations associated with strokes were included (US$541 versus US$947, p=0.02). However, the total mean hospital costs (US$1,854 versus US$1,834, p=0.96) and the total mean hospital costs plus physician costs (US$2,586 versus US$2,482, p=0.83) were similar in both groups.

8.1.3   From evidence to recommendations

Much of clinical practice in the management of paroxysmal AF has been based on relatively small trials of short duration in (mainly) symptomatic subjects. Most pharmacological studies of paroxysmal AF have concentrated on the reduction of symptomatic recurrences of paroxysmal AF, despite many having asymptomatic episodes. Many studies have also involved mixed populations with paroxysmal AF, paroxysmal atrial flutter or persistent AF.

Those patients who are asymptomatic or have rare paroxysms (eg only a few paroxysms a year) may decide not to take routine medication or to use a pill-in-the-pocket strategy, and the patient's views need to be considered. Similarly, where paroxysms are induced by precipitants (eg caffeine or alcohol), these need to be avoided by the patient, in which case treatment may not be necessary or a pill-in-the-pocket strategy could be adopted.

An escalating approach to drug therapy in paroxysmal AF could be recommended depending on the frequency of a patient's paroxysms and the need for increasingly effective antiarrhythmic drugs. For example, a beta-blocker could be prescribed in the first instance and in patients where this did not adequately control the paroxysms a Class Ic drug could be administered followed by amiodarone as a third-line option. This escalation of drug use is in the opposite direction of the evidence on efficacy alone as this did not fully cover the issue of the side effects (especially long-term) of the more efficacious agents.

Propafenone appeared to be at least as effective as sotalol in preventing the recurrence of AF for up to 12 months following administration,[134,187] although for longer periods propafenone was more effective.[136] The two drugs were comparable in terms of side effects.[187] It was noted that Class Ic agents (propafenone and flecainide) should be used with caution in patients with structural heart disease or coronary artery disease.

Amiodarone was more effective than sotalol[132,133] and propafenone[112] in the prevention of recurrent AF. Due to concerns regarding contraindications of Class Ic agents in patients with left ventricular dysfunction, amiodarone was regarded as the drug of choice in these patients with symptomatic paroxysms despite initial beta-blocker therapy.

The concerns over the long-term toxicity of amiodarone were not addressed in the evidence. Although the clinical evidence demonstrated that amiodarone was the most effective drug, its long-term use in patients with infrequent paroxysms needed to be fully weighed against the risk of side effects, especially since some (eg lung fibrosis) could be serious.

The advice given in the *British National Formulary* suggested that Class I and III agents should be administered under a hospital physician, but it was stressed that this did not necessarily mean that the patient had to be hospitalised and it was the decision to administer the drug that required the necessary expertise.

The evidence only addressed the suppression of paroxysms and did not cover the control of heart rate or the prevention of complications from paroxysmal AF (eg stroke). It was considered important that patients have their symptoms and medication reviewed regularly to determine whether a patient:

- had any side effects
- had a continued need for treatment
- could have their medication dose reduced.

It was also considered important that patients should not be left on medication long-term without review.

In terms of the cost of AF, amiodarone was cheaper than sotalol or propafenone, although this was based on a one-year follow-up study and costs of side effects may not have been adequately included in the analysis.

RECOMMENDATIONS

R27   Where patients have infrequent paroxysms and few symptoms, or where symptoms are induced by known precipitants (such as alcohol, caffeine), a 'no drug treatment' strategy or a pill-in-the-pocket strategy should be considered and discussed with the patient.   D(GPP)

R28   In patients with symptomatic paroxysms (with or without structural heart disease,* including coronary artery disease) a standard beta-blocker should be the initial treatment option.   D(GPP)

R29   In patients with paroxysmal AF and no structural heart disease:*
- where symptomatic suppression is not achieved with standard beta-blockers, either
  - a Class Ic agent (such as flecainide or propafenone), or   D(GPP)
  - sotalol**   D(GPP)

  should be given.
- where symptomatic suppression is not achieved with standard beta-blockers, Class Ic agents or sotalol, either
  - amiodarone, or   B
  - referral for non-pharmacological intervention (see section 12.3)

  should be considered.   A

R30   In patients with paroxysmal AF and coronary artery disease:
  - where standard beta-blockers do not achieve symptomatic suppression, sotalol should be given*   D(GPP)
  - where neither standard beta-blockers nor sotalol achieve symptomatic suppression, either
    - amiodarone, or   B
    - referral for non-pharmacological intervention (see section 12.3)   A
    should be considered.

R31   In patients with paroxysmal AF with poor left ventricular function:
  - where standard beta-blockers are given as part of the routine management strategy and adequately suppress paroxysms, no further treatment for paroxysms is needed   D(GPP)
  - where standard beta-blockers do not adequately suppress paroxysms, either
    - amiodarone or   B
    - referral for non-pharmacological intervention (see section 12.3)   A
    should be considered.

R32   Patients on long-term medication for paroxysmal AF should be kept under review to assess the need for continued treatment and the development of any adverse effects. D(GPP)

*Coronary artery disease or left ventricular dysfunction.
**Progressively titrated from 80 mg twice daily up to 240 mg twice daily.

8.2 Treatment strategy for paroxysmal AF

In selected patients with recurrent paroxysmal AF, out-of-hospital initiation of antiarrhythmic drugs may be possible, allowing for earlier treatment, a shorter duration of AF and a presumed likelihood of restoring and maintaining sinus rhythm. A pill-in-the-pocket approach is used in those not taking drugs regularly due to infrequent symptoms/paroxysms, or can be taken as an 'extra' drug dose in those already on a low maintenance of that particular drug. This approach is different to the out-of-hospital use of antiarrhythmic drugs in patients with recurrent persistent AF, where the aim may be to achieve pharmacological cardioversion *per se* or to improve the likelihood of subsequent elective electrical cardioversion (see Chapter 5), or to maintain sinus rhythm (see section 6.1).

The main concern with a pill-in-the-pocket approach is the risk of proarrhythmia often associated with antiarrhythmic drugs. Thus, the pill-in-the-pocket approach has generally been advocated only in those patients with a low risk of proarrhythmia and other adverse side effects. Such patients are typically those with no structural heart disease, absence of heart failure or left ventricular dysfunction, and where there is evidence that the antiarrhythmic drug used has previously worked successfully with no adverse effects (eg after at least one inpatient trial of the drug administered as a single oral dose, under ECG monitoring).

The antiarrhythmic drugs amiodarone and propafenone have both been considered in a number of trials comparing the safety and efficacy of a single oral dose of the drug with the intravenous administration of the same drug.[82–85] In all of these trials, patients were selected on the basis of relatively young age and the absence of any severe underlying structural heart disease. There was no incidence of ventricular proarrhythmia reported in either the intravenous or oral administration arms of these trials, and the incidence of successful cardioversion within 8 or 24 hours was comparable in most cases.

The objective of this section is to determine in which patients a single oral-dose antiarrhythmic drug may be safely used as a pill-in-the-pocket approach.

8.2.1 Methodological introduction

Studies were included if a comparison was made in terms of the safety, efficacy and impact on healthcare resources between the out-of-hospital self-administration of pharmacological cardioversion and the supervised, in-hospital administration in a well-defined patient cohort with either AF or supraventricular tachycardia (SVT). Studies were not included if the pharmacological agents were administered prophylactically.

Both of the included studies were based in Italy and compared the rates of hospital admission and emergency room treatment in a single cohort of patients in the period before and the period after the self-administration of antiarrhythmic drugs for the termination of either paroxysmal AF[190] or paroxysmal SVT.[191]

Neither study specified the treatment protocol during the period before the self-administration of antiarrhythmic drugs, or made a comparison between the two periods in terms of safety and efficacy.

8.2.2 Evidence statements

One study[190] found that the average number of admissions per month for emergency treatment was significantly lower during treatment of paroxysmal AF using a pill-in-the-pocket approach with Class Ic drugs than during conventional treatment (4.9 versus 45.6, p<0.001) in a population of patients with the following criteria: (2+)

* age 18 to 75
* left ventricular ejection fraction (LVEF) greater than 50%
* no history of severe heart disease
* systolic blood pressure (BP) greater than 100 mmHg
* heart rate greater than 70 bpm.

Another study found a similar result using similar selection criteria among patients with paroxysmal SVT.[191] (2+)

8.2.3 From evidence to recommendations

The limited evidence suggested that pill-in-the-pocket treatment was associated with a lower incidence of inpatient and emergency hospital admissions than conventional treatment.[190,191] It was uncertain whether the pill-in-the-pocket strategy was associated with more adverse events, or reduced episode duration when compared to in-hospital treatment.

Within the UK, the number of patients managed in this way is currently thought to be small, and patients need to be made more aware of this treatment option, although strict selection criteria are deemed necessary. In particular, it was considered that patient education in its use is vital.

Therapy for paroxysmal AF should be tailored to the patient. For example, episodes of AF for 1 to 2 minutes once a year or for 10 hours twice a day are both paroxysmal AF, but their impact on the patient's quality of life, if symptomatic, would be quite different. In patients with infrequent and brief paroxysms, the regular use of antiarrhythmic therapy may not be necessary (and is commonly not prescribed in current clinical practice). Such patients may be suitable for the pill-in-the-pocket approach. However, for infrequent but protracted and symptomatic paroxysmal AF, rapid cardioversion of each event and/or antiarrhythmic drug prophylaxis may be considered.

RECOMMENDATION

R33   In patients with paroxysmal AF, a pill-in-the-pocket strategy should be considered in those who:

- have no history of left ventricular dysfunction, or valvular or ischaemic heart disease; and
- have a history of infrequent symptomatic episodes of paroxysmal AF; and
- have a systolic blood pressure greater than 100 mm Hg and a resting heart rate above 70 bpm; and
- are able to understand how to, and when to, take the medication.   C

8.3   Antithrombotic therapy for paroxysmal AF

Patients with paroxysmal AF appear to carry the same risk of stroke and thromboembolism as those with persistent AF.[192] Whether the risk is dependent upon the frequency of the paroxysms or their duration is unclear.[193] In addition, patients frequently get asymptomatic paroxysms[31] and may still be at risk of thromboembolism. There is evidence of some clustering of thromboembolic events around the time of onset of AF[167,194] and following successful cardioversion.[139] Compared with permanent AF, patients with paroxysmal AF tend to be younger[18] and have a lower prevalence of associated clinical risk factors.

8.3.1   Methodological introduction

No studies were found that considered the efficacy of antithrombotic therapy compared with placebo in a population comprising only paroxysmal AF patients.

However, subgroups of patients with paroxysmal AF were reported in two meta-analyses. One meta-analysis[192] pooled data from the aspirin treatment arms of three serial trials and compared ischaemic stroke rates in the paroxysmal AF subgroup with those of non-paroxysmal AF patients. The second study[174] compared the effects of anticoagulation and antiplatelet therapy on rates of ischaemic stroke and major bleeding in a subgroup of participants with paroxysmal AF.

8.3.2 Evidence statements

One meta-analysis[174] found that in patients treated with aspirin, the incidence of stroke was similar in those with paroxysmal AF and those with non-paroxysmal AF. (2++)

One meta-analysis[192] found adjusted-dose warfarin to be associated with a reduced incidence of ischaemic stroke compared with aspirin (1.5% versus 4.7%, respectively, p<0.05), although no significant difference was found in terms of the incidence of bleeding events. The study also found the efficacy of warfarin in reducing the incidence of stroke to be comparable between those with paroxysmal and those with non-paroxysmal AF. (1+)

8.3.3 From evidence to recommendations

The data from clinical trials were limited by the relatively small number of patients with paroxysmal AF (approximately 12% of subjects in five randomised trials).[192] There was some evidence that patients with paroxysmal AF receiving aspirin experience a similar rate of ischaemic stroke as patients with non-paroxysmal AF who receive aspirin.[192]

The effectiveness of anticoagulation compared with antiplatelet therapy in reducing the rate of ischaemic stroke is similar for patients with either paroxysmal AF or non-paroxysmal AF.[174] The rate of adverse bleeding events associated with anticoagulation is also similar between the two groups.[174]

In current clinical practice, the indicators for antithrombotic therapy are highly variable (often depending on the clinical presentation of symptoms). For example, the more frequent a patient's paroxysms the more likely they will be prescribed anticoagulants, despite the risk of stroke being determined by the presence of associated risk factors. It was concluded that patients with paroxysmal AF required a similar degree of anticoagulation as patients with permanent AF, but that further studies would be required to confirm this.

RECOMMENDATION

R34 Decisions on the need for antithrombotic therapy in patients with paroxysmal AF should not be based on the frequency or duration of paroxysms (symptomatic or asymptomatic) but on appropriate risk stratification, as for permanent AF (see section 11.6).   B

8.4   Rhythm-control treatment algorithm for paroxysmal AF

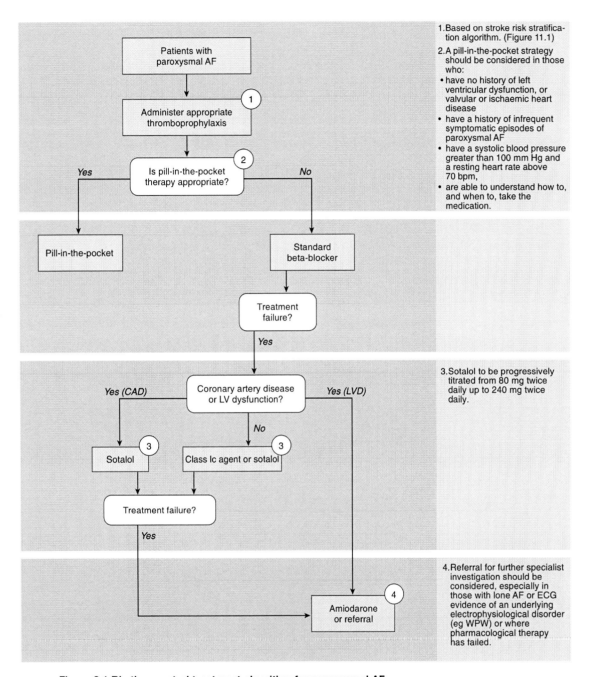

Figure 8.1 Rhythm-control treatment algorithm for paroxysmal AF

9 | Treatment for acute-onset AF

9.1 Acute AF in haemodynamically unstable patients

Although most patients in AF present without haemodynamic compromise, there is a small group of patients who are significantly compromised by the onset of AF. These patients require immediate hospitalisation and urgent intervention to prevent further deterioration.

Those considered at highest risk from haemodynamic instability caused by AF have been defined as:[195]

- those with a ventricular rate greater than 150 bpm
- ongoing chest pain, or
- critical perfusion.

In these circumstances, the concerns regarding intervention in the absence of anticoagulation and echocardiography are counterbalanced by the need for urgent treatment. This may include the need to treat important problems such as hypoxia, left ventricular failure, acute ischaemia, pyrexia and electrolyte disorders.

A number of specific issues are recognised in current UK practice for the management of patients with AF in the presence of haemodynamic instability:[65]

- The slow onset of digoxin makes it inappropriate for use in this situation.
- Patients whose AF is associated with thyrotoxicosis will not respond to any strategy that does not first treat the underlying thyroid disease.
- Patients with an accessory pathway such as Wolff–Parkinson–White (WPW) syndrome are particularly at risk following the onset of AF because they can present with high ventricular rates (greater than 200 bpm) and may need specific management.

Treatment with AV node blockers (eg adenosine, digoxin, verapamil, diltiazem) will unmask or exacerbate a rapid AF due to a WPW syndrome and are therefore contraindicated in such patients.[196]

In patients with AF associated with an unacceptably high ventricular rate the primary aim is one of rate control. In other patients with acceptable ventricular rates whose cardiac function has been compromised by AF onset in the context of other cardiac abnormalities (eg hypertensive heart disease, valvular heart disease), rate control is unlikely to bring about clinical improvement and there is a need for the restoration of sinus rhythm.

In clinical practice, amiodarone is the most common agent used in the management of patients presenting in AF with haemodynamic compromise, as it appears to have a hybrid effect of rapid reduction in ventricular rate in most patients with a proportion of these reverting to sinus rhythm over a longer period. An alternative choice suitable for use in patients with invasive monitoring is esmolol, which is an intravenous beta-blocker with a short half-life, which allows for accurate and frequent titration.

9.1.1 Methodological introduction

No studies were found that made a direct comparison between different treatment strategies in haemodynamically unstable patients. However, one observational study[26] was found reporting outcomes between different emergency interventions for AF. This study was in a mixed population including haemodynamically stable patients, and excluded those in whom immediate electrical cardioversion (ECV) or intubation was indicated on the basis of severe haemodynamic instability or respiratory failure. Nonetheless, the mean ventricular rate reported in this study did suggest the presence of rapid AF in a substantial proportion of the included patients.

In addition, three other studies were found reporting the effectiveness of either diltiazem in the acute control of ventricular rate[197] or amiodarone for acute pharmacological cardioversion[112,198] in patients with rapid AF.

Only one study[198] was found in the context of severe haemodynamic instability, occurring in an intensive-care setting in ventilated patients with severely impaired left ventricular dysfunction.

No studies were found reporting the effectiveness of ECV in the successful treatment of AF in the context of haemodynamic instability, although one study[26] did report the effectiveness of ECV in a population consisting primarily of acute-onset AF patients with a fast ventricular rate and a previous attempt at pharmacological cardioversion (PCV).

Studies that considered head-to-head drug comparisons for either ventricular rate-control or PCV are not considered here. For a comparison of drugs for use in PCV, see section 5.2 above; for use in ventricular rate control see section 7.1 above.

9.1.2 Evidence statements

One observational study[26] found that ECV successfully restored sinus rhythm in 89% of patients presenting with acute-onset AF and a mean ventricular rate of 122 bpm. Eighty-three per cent were refractory to an earlier attempt at pharmacological cardioversion using procainamide (which was successful in 50% of cases at doses between 500 and 1000 mg and had an incidence of adverse events of 9%).[28] The study reported no complications associated with ECV.[28]

Three studies[198–200] found the intravenous administration of amiodarone (eg 5 mg/kg over 5 minutes) to be an effective treatment for the restoration of sinus rhythm in patients with varying degrees of haemodynamic instability, including a group of intubated patients with severely impaired cardiac function.[28,198] However, one study[199] found an increased risk of bradycardia following amiodarone in those presenting with a slower initial heart rate. (2+)

One study[26] found the administration of rate-controlling drugs (beta-blockers, rate-limiting calcium antagonists or digoxin) to be an effective strategy to reduce ventricular rate in 75% of AF patients with a fast ventricular rate.[28] A similar result was reported in another study[197] with the rate-limiting calcium antagonist diltiazem.[28]

Two studies[198,200] found the intravenous administration of amiodarone (5 mg/kg over 3 to 5 minutes[200] or 300 mg bolus via central line[198]) to be an effective strategy to control ventricular rate in haemodynamically impaired patients.[28]

9.1.3 From evidence to recommendations

Based on limited available evidence, pharmacological rate-control and both pharmacological and electrical cardioversion are effective treatment options for the acute management of patients presenting with various degrees of haemodynamic instability.

In UK clinical practice, very sick patients with fast AF and haemodynamic compromise were often inappropriately administered iv flecainide. Flecainide should not be used in such patients unless they are known to have rapid AF consequent upon a WPW syndrome.

It was noted that the use of AV node blockers would unmask or exacerbate a rapid AF due to a WPW syndrome and their use is contraindicated in these patients. Digoxin was less effective in haemodynamically compromised patients due to its slow onset of action and possible adrenergic activity.

Intravenous amiodarone is widely used as it both rapidly reduces ventricular heart rate and cardioverts AF. In an emergency setting, amiodarone is likely to be administered intravenously via a peripheral line.

RECOMMENDATIONS

R35   In patients with a life-threatening deterioration in haemodynamic stability following the onset of AF, emergency electrical cardioversion should be performed, irrespective of the duration of the AF.   D

R36   In patients with non life-threatening haemodynamic instability following the onset of AF:
- electrical cardioversion should be performed   D
- where there is a delay in organising electrical cardioversion, intravenous amiodarone should be used   D
- in those with known Wolff–Parkinson–White syndrome:
    - flecainide may be used as an alternative for attempting pharmacological cardioversion
    - atrioventricular node-blocking agents (such as diltiazem, verapamil or digoxin) should not be used.   D(GPP)

R37   In patients with known permanent AF where haemodynamic instability is caused mainly by a poorly controlled ventricular rate, a pharmacological rate-control strategy should be used.   D

R38   Where urgent pharmacological rate-control is indicated, intravenous treatment should be with one of the following:
- beta-blockers or rate-limiting calcium antagonists   D
- amiodarone, where beta-blockers or calcium antagonists are contraindicated or ineffective.   D

9.2 Antithrombotic therapy for acute-onset AF

The aim of this section is to examine which antithrombotic therapy, if any, is most effective in treating patients with acute-onset AF, including the postoperative setting.

The onset of AF is associated with a cluster of thromboembolic events,[167] but the development of intra-atrial thrombi, and the immediate risk of thromboembolism, is perceived to be minimal within the first 48 hours.

In one study of 357 patients with symptomatic acute-onset AF of less than 48 hour duration (of whom 250 converted spontaneously to sinus rhythm and 107 underwent cardioversion without any anticoagulation), thromboembolism only occurred in three patients.[140] In another series of 258 patients undergoing cardioversion for AF of less than 2 days duration, only one embolic event occurred out of 198 patients who did not receive pre- or post-cardioversion warfarin.[143] However, in a further study, patients with acute AF of an apparent duration of less than 3 days were found to have an intra-atrial thrombus detected by TOE in approximately 15% of cases.[201] This raises the possibilities that either the development of intra-atrial thrombus may be more rapid than previously suspected and/or that some cases of presumed recent-onset AF may have had the arrhythmia (possibly asymptomatically) for longer.

Thus, in patients presenting *de novo* with AF, a clear history of arrhythmia onset is necessary in order to guide appropriate antithrombotic therapy and, if performed, the safety of cardioversion.

9.2.1 Methodological introduction

No studies were found that addressed this clinical area.

9.2.2 From evidence to recommendations

Although no randomised trials have specifically addressed the issue of acute-onset AF, common clinical practice indicates that cardioversion may be safely performed without the need for oral anticoagulation if AF has been present for less than 48 hours.[202] However, in cases of uncertainty about arrhythmia onset, anticoagulation therapy is warranted.

The GDG discussed the use of intravenous unfractionated heparin and subcutaneous low molecular weight heparin (LMWH). Both drugs are routinely used in clinical practice in the acute and peri-cardioversion periods. It was agreed that anticoagulation with heparin could be started at the presentation of acute AF while the INR remains subtherapeutic during the initiating phase of oral anticoagulation.

Acute AF may present with a fast ventricular response, leading to haemodynamic instability, which may require urgent direct current (DC) cardioversion. Where the degree of haemodynamic instability is life threatening (for example, cardiogenic shock), DC cardioversion may need to be performed rapidly and in such cases would take priority over the need for anticoagulation.

RECOMMENDATIONS

R39   In patients with acute AF who are receiving no, or subtherapeutic, anticoagulation
        therapy: D(GPP)

    • in the absence of contraindications, heparin should be started at initial presentation
    • heparin should be continued until a full assessment has been made and appropriate
      antithrombotic therapy has been started, based on risk stratification (see section 11.6).

R40   In patients with a confirmed diagnosis of acute AF of recent onset (less than 48 hours since
        onset), oral anticoagulation should be used if:

    • stable sinus rhythm is not successfully restored within the same 48-hour period following
      onset of acute AF, or
    • there are factors indicating a high risk of AF recurrence,* or
    • it is recommended by the stroke risk stratification algorithm (see Figure 11.1).   D(GPP)

R41   In patients with acute AF where there is uncertainty over the precise time since onset,
        oral anticoagulation should be used, as for persistent AF (see section 6.2).   D(GPP)

R42   In cases of acute AF where the patient is haemodynamically unstable, any emergency
        intervention should be performed as soon as possible and the initiation of
        anticoagulation should not delay any emergency intervention.   D(GPP)

*Factors indicating a high risk of AF recurrence include:
    • a history of failed attempts at cardioversion
    • structural heart disease (mitral valve disease, left ventricular dysfunction or an enlarged left atrium)
    • a prolonged history of AF (greater than 12 months)
    • previous recurrences of AF.

9.3 Haemodynamically unstable AF treatment algorithm

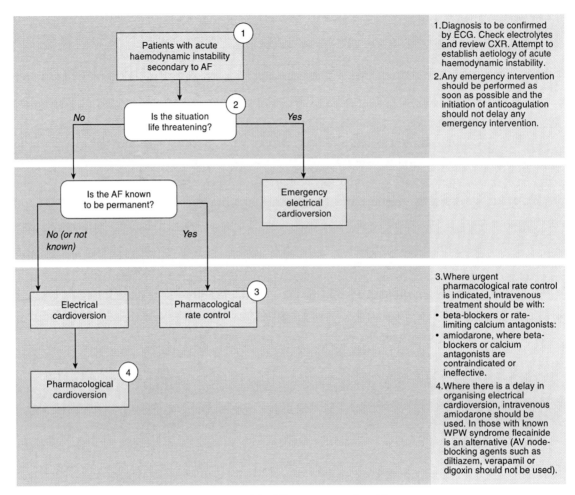

Figure 9.1 Haemodynamically unstable AF treatment algorithm

10 | Postoperative AF

Postoperative AF (post-op AF) following cardiothoracic surgery is a significant problem, occurring in approximately 33% of patients after coronary heart surgery.[203] The occurrence following valvular heart surgery is even higher.[204]

Post-op AF is associated with a greater risk of mortality and morbidity.[205] Evidence is also emerging[206] that post-op AF predisposes people to a significantly increased risk of stroke and thromboembolism, suggesting that patients should be anticoagulated where post-op AF persists for more than 48 hours.[207]

Although post-op AF can be transient and generally self-limiting, treatment is indicated for those patients who remain symptomatic, become haemodynamically unstable, and develop cardiac ischaemia or heart failure. Conventional treatment strategies have included ECV, atrial overdrive pacing using temporary epicardial pacing leads (if atrial flutter is the dominant rhythm), pharmacological rate control and antithrombotic therapy. Cardioversion may also be attempted prior to hospital discharge.

Management of medical comorbidities (eg hypoxia) and the correction of underlying electrolyte imbalance (especially potassium and magnesium) is well recognised[208,209] in the prevention of post-op AF. Most units have strategies to maintain the serum potassium above 4 mmol per litre and some will often endeavour to maintain the serum potassium higher than 4.5 mmol per litre.[210] One recent meta-analysis[211] found that magnesium administration is an effective prophylactic measure for the prevention of post-op AF, but did not significantly alter length of stay or in-hospital mortality.

Currently, there is significant variation in the management of post-op AF. The aim of this chapter is to assess whether the perioperative administration of antiarrhythmic drugs is effective prophylaxis to prevent post-op AF (section 10.1), and in those cases where post-op AF develops, to determine which is the most effective treatment strategy (section 10.2).

10.1 Drug prophylaxis for postoperative AF

10.1.1 Methodological introduction

Of the studies considering prophylaxis, the majority concerned the prevention of post-op AF following cardiac surgery, and most of these results are summarised in a meta-analysis.[212] The other studies[213–218] considered non-cardiac thoracic procedures (eg pneumonectomy).

The reporting of side effects associated with antiarrhythmic drugs was not consistent, with many studies having too few participants to make any meaningful comparisons.

Studies were included if comparison was made between an antiarrhythmic drug or cardiac glycoside available in the UK, and a placebo or no-treatment control. The management of electrolyte imbalance (eg magnesium or potassium) was not assessed.

Five US studies[218,219–222] considering the cost-effectiveness of drug prophylaxis were appraised and met quality criteria.

- Two studies[219,220] estimated the mean cost per case of post-op AF avoided, of oral amiodarone prophylaxis versus no prophylaxis in patients undergoing coronary bypass grafting (CABG).
- One study[221] estimated the cost per AF averted of intravenous amiodarone therapy in CABG, valve and CABG plus valve patients, according to their predicted risk of postoperative AF.
- One study[218] estimated the median total hospital costs in patients with and without oral amiodarone prophylaxis based on the medical records of patients after pulmonary resection.
- One study[222] estimated the total hospitalisation costs in a RCT of oral amiodarone prophylaxis versus placebo in patients undergoing cardiopulmonary bypass.
- One study[219] estimated the total hospital costs in oral amiodarone prophylaxis versus placebo groups based on the Atrial Fibrillation Suppression Trial.

10.1.2 Evidence statements

▷   Drug prophylaxis in cardiac surgery

Amiodarone

In a meta-analysis of 14 studies[212] which compared amiodarone with placebo or no treatment, amiodarone administered pre-, intra- or postoperatively was found to be associated with a reduced incidence of post-op AF or other supraventricular arrhythmia (OR 0.54, 95% CI 0.44 to 0.67; $p<0.00001$) (1+). Similar results were found in other primary studies.[223–230] (1++)

In one study[231] amiodarone was significantly associated with a reduced incidence of post-op AF lasting longer than 24 hours, and episodes that required treatment, compared with placebo. (1++)

One study[224] found that amiodarone resulted in a reduced duration of post-op AF compared with no treatment (11.0 versus 16.2 days; $p<0.001$) (2+). Two smaller studies[222,232] found no significant difference in the duration of post-op AF. (1++)

One study[231] found rapid preoperative amiodarone loading resulted in more nausea than placebo (31.3% versus 16.0%; $p=0.018$), this was not observed with slow loading (21.4% versus 16.0%) (1++). There was no difference reported in the incidence of hypotension for either strategy. (1++)

Beta-blockers (excluding sotalol)

One meta-analysis of 28 studies[212] found beta-blockers (excluding sotalol) resulted in less post-op AF and other supraventricular arrhythmias (OR 0.35, 95% CI 0.26 to 0.49; $p<0.00001$) (1+). This result is consistent with the results of other primary studies,[226,230,233–235] in one of which[226] there was a significant increase in postoperative symptomatic bradycardia (less than 40 bpm) compared with placebo (16.1% versus 3.1%; $p<0.05$). (1+)

Sotalol

A meta-analysis of eight studies[212] found sotalol reduced post-op AF and other supraventricular arrhythmias compared with control (OR 0.36, 95% CI 0.23 to 0.56) (1+). Two other primary studies[226,236] showed similar results, one of which[226] found a significant association between the use of sotalol (240 mg three times a day) and the incidence of postoperative symptomatic bradycardia (<40 bpm) compared with placebo (12.7% versus 3.1%; p<0.05) (1+). The study did not report any incidence of pro-arrhythmic side effects associated with sotalol.

Rate-limiting calcium antagonists

Four studies[237–240] found the rate-limiting calcium antagonist diltiazem to be significantly associated with a lower incidence of post-op AF compared with placebo or no treatment (1++). A similar result has also been found for the rate-limiting calcium antagonist verapamil.[241] (1+)

Propafenone

One study[242] found propafenone administered at 675 mg/day (although not at 450 mg/day) decreased post-op AF compared with placebo. (1++)

Procainamide

One study[243] found no difference in the incidence of post-op AF between procainamide and placebo but did reduce the number of patient days spent in post-op AF (16 versus 19 days; p<0.05) (1++). It was found to be significantly associated with an increased incidence of nausea compared with placebo (64% versus 32%; p<0.01) (1++). Another smaller study[244] (N=46) found procainamide to be significantly associated with a reduced incidence of post-op AF compared with placebo (3.9% versus 10.6%; p<0.04). (1++)

Digoxin

A meta-analysis of two studies,[235] as well as another primary study[245] not included in the meta-analysis found digoxin did not reduce post-op AF when compared with no treatment. (1+)

▷ Drug prophylaxis in thoracic (non-cardiac) surgery

Beta-blockers

One study[246] found beta-blockers to be effective in reducing post-op AF compared with placebo in favour of beta-blockers (6.7% versus 40.0%; p<0.05) (1+). Another[217] found a non-significant reduction in any arrhythmia requiring treatment but increased incidences of post-operative bradycardia and hypotension respectively (25% versus 4% compared with placebo; p=0.018; 49% versus 26% compared with placebo; p=0.003). (1++)

Rate-limiting calcium antagonists

One study[213] found diltiazem did not significantly reduce the overall incidence of post-op AF; but when considering those over 60 years old only (15% versus 25%; p=0.05), or when other cardiac arrhythmias were included (14% versus 26%; p=0.03), diltiazem was effective (1++). Another study[214] did not find diltiazem effective compared with placebo (8% versus 15%). (1+)

Flecainide

One study[215] found flecainide effectively reduced all postoperative cardiac arrhythmia requiring treatment (including AF) compared with placebo (0% versus 6%; p<0.05). (1++)

Digoxin

One study[216] found no other treatments compared with digoxin in reducing the incidence of post-op AF following pneumonectomy (31% versus 28%). (2+)

Amiodarone

One study[218] found amiodarone reduced post-op AF compared with no treatment (9.7% versus 33%; p=0.025) following pneumonectomy. (2+)

Health economics

There was no significant difference in total hospital costs in oral amiodarone prophylaxis versus placebo (US$15,565 + US$9,832 versus US$16,126 + US$8,043, p=0.12) and a higher percent of episodes of AF prevented (77% versus 62%).[219]

There was no significant difference between median total hospital costs (US$30,800 (20,400–96,900) in 50 patients without prophylaxis versus US$26,700 (11,000–55,900) in 31 patients with low dose oral amiodarone prophylaxis). Significantly less patients developed postoperative AF with low dose oral amiodarone (9.7% versus 33%, p=0.0253).[218]

One study[222] found a significantly lower mean total cost of hospitalisation in the oral amiodarone group compared with placebo in patients undergoing cardiopulmonary bypass surgery (US$18, 375 + US$13,863 versus US$26,491 + US$23,837, p=0.03).

One study[219,220] estimated the mean cost per AF event avoided was lower in the oral amiodarone group versus no prophylaxis (US$15,750, 95% CI US$15,591 to US$15,999 versus US$17,426, 95% CI US$17,252 to US$17,600). Multivariate sensitivity analysis indicated these findings were most sensitive to the cost of hospitalisation and frequency of AF.

One study[221] indicated the cost effectiveness of prophylactic intravenous amiodarone therapy varied according to the type of cardiac surgery and predicted risk of postoperative AF. As the risk of AF in the targeted patients increases, the cost-effectiveness ratio improves.

- For CABG patients, the ICERs ranged from US$10,938 for the highest risk patients to US$55,854 per AF averted in the lowest risk patients.
- For valve replacement patients the ICERs ranged from US$4,219 in the highest risk patients to US$43,011 per AF averted in the lowest risk patients.
- For CABG and valve replacement patients the ICERs ranged from US$69 for the highest risk patients to US$39,698 per AF averted in the lowest risk patients.

10.1.3 From evidence to recommendations

Although no specific evidence was evaluated regarding the association between electrolyte balance and the incidence of post-op AF, it was agreed that scrupulous attention to electrolyte balance was important.

Drug prophylaxis to reduce the risk of post-op AF relates to the need to:

- continue existing medication (eg beta-blockers)
- administer a drug preoperatively (eg beta-blockers or amiodarone), or
- administer a drug in the immediate postoperative period (eg sotalol or amiodarone).

In many of the studies, the majority of patients were already taking beta-blockers preoperatively, and these were either discontinued in the postoperative period or continued, despite the use of beta-blockers being recognised as an independent (negative) predictor of post-op AF.[247,248] In those studies where beta-blockers were continued postoperatively, the results may be confounded by this additional cardioprotective effect, which may be insensitive to additional antiarrhythmic medication, particularly beta-blockers, thus underestimating the effectiveness of the prophylaxis.

Alternatively, in those studies where beta-blockers were discontinued, the incidence of post-op AF may be exaggerated by the withdrawal of the cardioprotective effects of beta-blockers, which in some patients may have been preventing the development of arrhythmias aetiologically independent from post-op AF.

For non-cardiac thoracic surgery, there was evidence for efficacy of the same drugs as used in cardiac surgery in the prevention of post-op AF.

It was agreed that beta-blockers, including sotalol, were effective prophylactic drugs, and that those patients who were receiving pre-existing therapy with these drugs would benefit from a reduced risk of post-op AF if those drugs were continued, unless there were compelling reasons to withdraw them (eg postoperative hypotension or bradycardia).

It was agreed that digoxin is not effective in preventing postoperative AF.[235,245]

Administering amiodarone slowly over 5 to 7 days preoperatively and continuing during the perioperative period is more effective and associated with fewer side effects than more rapid loading.[231]

There is an increased risk of bradycardia associated with the use of beta-blockers and nausea associated with procainamide, as well as with amiodarone when loaded rapidly in the preoperative period.

Data from the USA suggest the prophylactic administration of amiodarone for the prevention of post-op AF is cost effective, particularly in high-risk patients, compared with no prophylaxis for certain cardiac procedures. It was noted that there may be cost differentials between the UK and the USA for antiarrhythmic drugs.

RECOMMENDATIONS

R43   In the prophylaxis and management of postoperative AF, the appropriate use of antithrombotic therapy and correction of identifiable precipitants (such as electrolyte imbalance or hypoxia) is recommended.   **D(GPP)**

R44   In patients undergoing cardiothoracic surgery:
- the risk of postoperative AF should be reduced by the administration of one of the following:
  - amiodarone   **A**
  - a beta-blocker   **A**
  - sotalol   **A**
  - a rate-limiting calcium antagonist   **B**
- digoxin should not be used.   **B**

R45   In patients undergoing cardiac surgery on pre-existing beta-blocker therapy, this treatment should be continued unless contraindications develop (such as postoperative bradycardia or hypotension).   **A**

10.2 Treatment for postoperative AF

10.2.1 Methodological introduction

The results of nine studies considering the treatment of postoperative AF were included, all except one[249] were prospective RCTs. The other was placebo-controlled[250] with a 2 × 2 crossover study design with no reported wash-out period between crossover. Of the reported RCTs, none had the statistical power to identify effect sizes that may be considered clinically significant.

A rate-control strategy was defined as one which involved the administration of drugs to control heart rate; a rhythm-control strategy was defined as one which involved treatment with electrical or pharmacological cardioversion or the administration of drugs known to be effective in pharmacological cardioversion. In many studies the objectives of each treatment group were not explicitly reported, in which case a comparison of a rate-control treatment strategy with a rhythm-control treatment strategy was presumed based on the established differential actions of the interventions considered. The duration of follow-up times varied between the studies (less than 1 hour to 30 days).

One study[250] compared rhythm control to no-treatment. All of the other studies compared rate control with pharmacological rhythm control. There were no studies comparing either rate control with rhythm control using electrical cardioversion or rate control versus no treatment.

None of the studies reported results for patients with post-op AF and haemodynamic instability requiring urgent medical intervention.

10.2.2 Evidence statements

In patients with post-op AF, where various rhythm- and rate-control strategies have been compared (see Tables 10.1 and 10.2), rhythm control results in:

- greater cardioversion within 1 hour but not after 24 hours[250–255]
- shorter time for restoration of sinus rhythm[256]
- no difference in ventricular rate control[250,255]
- higher rates of therapeutic effectiveness[255]
- no difference in relapse rates.[256]

Table 10.1 Comparison of rhythm-control treatments for post-op AF with rate-controlling treatments or no treatment in terms of percentage of patients reverting to sinus rhythm

	Comparison	N	Period (hours)	Rhythm (%)	Control (%)	p
(1+)	Flecainide/digoxin[255]	29	1	60	0	<0.001
(1+)	Propafenone/placebo[250]	14	1	43	0	<0.001
(1+)	Procainamide/digoxin[252]	30	12	93	60	<0.05
(1+)	Sotalol/digoxin*[253]	40	12	85	85	NS
(1+)	Propafenone/various**[251]	32	24	35	50	NS
(1+)	Amiodarone/digoxin[254]	30	24	93	87	NS

*Digoxin with additional disopyramide if sinus rhythm was not restored within 2 hours.
**Various = uncontrolled use of beta-blockers, calcium antagonists or digoxin in both treatment arms.

Table 10.2 Comparison of rhythm-control treatments for post-op AF with rate-controlling treatments or no treatment

	Outcome	N	Test/control	Test	Control	p
(1+)	Conversion time, hours	50	Rhythm-control drugs/ rate-control drugs*[256]	11.2	11.8	NS
(1+)	Therapeutic rate control	24	Propafenone/no treatment[250]	26%	2%	<000.1
(1+)	Therapeutic rate control**	29	Flecainide/digoxin[255]	7%	14%	NS
(1+)	Therapeutic effectiveness	29	Flecainide/digoxin[255]	67%	14%	<0.001
(1+)	AF recurrence at 1 week	50	Rhythm-control drugs/ rate control drugs*[256]	24%	28%	NS
(1+)	AF recurrence at 4 weeks	50	Rhythm-control drugs/ rate-control drugs*[256]	6%	12%	NS
(1+)	AF recurrence at 8 weeks	50	Rhythm-control drugs/ rate-control drugs*[256]	4%	9%	NS
(1+)	AF recurrence	40	Sotalol/digoxin†[253]	5%	35%	<0.05

*Rhythm-control drugs: sotalol, procainamide, propafenone or amiodarone.
Rate-control drugs: diltiazem, verapamil, beta-blockers or digoxin.
**HR <100 bpm within 45 minutes of administration.
†Digoxin with additional disopyramide if sinus rhythm was not restored within 2 hours.

Two studies[249,256] of various rhythm-control versus rate-control strategies have shown shorter overall length of hospital stay with rhythm-control strategies but results for postoperative length of stay have been inconsistent (see Table 10.3).

	Table 10.3 Comparison of rhythm-control and rate-control treatments in terms of length of stay (days)					
	Study	**N**	**LOS measure**	**Rhythm**	**Rate**	**p**
(1+)	Lee et al[256]	50	Hospital	9.0	13.2	<0.05
(1+)	Lee et al[256]	50	Post-op only	7.4	9.7	<0.01
(2+)	Shah et al[249]	101	Post-op only	8.3	6.3	<0.01

LOS measure = length of hospital stay measure.

10.2.3 From evidence to recommendations

The GDG agreed that the evidence suggested a trend towards a strategy of rhythm control over rate control. The evidence suggested that rhythm control produced a decreased time to cardioversion, prolonged maintenance of cardioversion, and decreased length of overall hospital stay.[256]

However, the data supported the use of a rhythm-control strategy in achieving sinus rhythm only in the short term. In the longer term, there is little difference in the maintenance of sinus rhythm between either strategy.[250–255] It was noted that the number of study participants was relatively small and the follow-up periods were relatively short. Overall, it was concluded that a rhythm-control strategy provided short-term benefits.

RECOMMENDATIONS

R46   Unless contraindicated, a rhythm-control strategy should be the initial management
        option for the treatment of postoperative AF following cardiothoracic surgery.   C

R47   Unless contraindicated, postoperative AF following non-cardiothoracic surgery
        should be managed as for acute-onset AF with any other precipitant.   D(GPP)

11 Antithrombotic therapy

11.1 Initiating antithrombotic therapy

AF is an independent predictor of stroke, with an annual risk that is 5 to 6 times higher than patients in sinus rhythm. However, this risk is not homogeneous, ranging from an annual risk of 1% in patients aged over 65 years old with no risk factors, to over 12% per year in patients who have a history of prior stroke, transient ischaemic attack or thromboembolism. Not only is AF a major risk factor for stroke, but when strokes occur in association with AF, the patients suffer substantial mortality, morbidity, disability and longer hospital stays compared with stroke patients without AF.

The benefits of thromboprophylaxis in patients with AF are well established in randomised trials, and most guidelines recommend the use of anticoagulation with warfarin for high-risk patients. However, there continues to be wide variation in management. In particular, the elderly are at the highest risk of stroke, and would benefit most from thromboprophylaxis. However, the elderly have more comorbidities and concomitant therapies that may preclude anticoagulant therapy. Also, most of the evidence on thromboprophylaxis has been based on hospital-managed populations and the application to primary care management and anticoagulation monitoring is still uncertain.

Common practice upon detection or initial presentation of a patient with AF in the community or when an AF patient presents to a non-specialist is to refer to a specialist clinic to decide on appropriate antithrombotic therapy. For example, in a survey of accident and emergency consultants in the UK, many were reluctant to make a decision regarding anticoagulation, and preferred referral to a medical or cardiology team.[257]

This may lead to delays in the institution of appropriate thromboprophylaxis, and may increase a patient's risk of stroke or thromboembolism. However, risk stratification for thromboprophylaxis can be easily performed on clinical criteria (see section 11.6).

Evidence-based guidance is required to determine whether it is beneficial to start antithrombotic therapy immediately following the initial diagnosis of AF, rather then delay initiation, pending assessment at a specialist clinic.

11.1.1 Methodological introduction

The literature search and evidence appraisal processes for this question resulted in no studies suitable for appraisal.

11.1.2 From evidence to recommendations

Although there was no appraisable evidence base, the issue of early versus delayed administration of anticoagulation in acute patients newly diagnosed with AF was considered of great importance. It was agreed that the administration of anticoagulation after treating comorbidities (eg hypertension) was good clinical practice.

RECOMMENDATION

R48   In patients with newly diagnosed AF for whom antithrombotic therapy is indicated
        (see section 11.6), such treatment should be initiated with minimal delay after the
        appropriate management of comorbidities.   D(GPP)

11.2 Antithrombotic therapy in acute stroke patients*

Approximately a third of patients presenting with an acute stroke are found to have AF. These
patients have high mortality and morbidity. Prior to the administration of antithrombotic
therapy, intracranial haemorrhage needs to be excluded, and an assessment of the risk from
haemorrhagic transformation in patients with large cerebral infarcts needs to be made. While
warfarin is superior to aspirin for the secondary prevention of stroke in AF,[258] there is
uncertainty about the optimal timing of administration of anticoagulants following acute
stroke. The presumption is that most of these patients have cardiogenic embolism, from
intracardiac thrombi, but many patients with AF can also develop lacunar strokes secondary to
hypertension and other comorbidities and in such cases warfarin is less effective.[259]

The mortality benefits of aspirin therapy following acute stroke[260] are less marked among
patients with AF. This may be due to the embolisation of pre-formed intra-atrial thrombus
rather than newly formed platelet-thrombus adhering to carotid and cerebral artery atheroma,
or may be a reflection of a lesser role of platelets in AF-related stroke.

The purpose of this section is to determine the most appropriate antithrombotic therapy – if
any – during the acute post-stroke phase, considering the efficacy of antithrombotic therapies
to reduce recurrent stroke, as well as the increased risk of intracranial haemorrhage (ICH) and
other major bleeding events.

11.2.1 Methodological introduction

One systematic review[260] considered the results of three primary trials. The trials included peri-
stroke patients of varying aetiology. The included studies reported a mean time to treatment of
between 19 and 25 hours. Data regarding the subgroup with AF had been published or made
available to the authors of the review. All the evidence statements are derived solely from the
subgroup comparisons of AF patients.

No trials involving warfarin or any other oral antithrombotic treatment for the prevention of
acute recurrent stroke were found.

One of the primary studies included in the systematic review was of a Chinese population.

11.2.2 Evidence statements

In patients with AF the incidence of acute recurrent ischaemic stroke was comparable between
treatment with LMWH and aspirin.[260] Another trial found a significant association when

---

*NICE is developing a clinical guideline on the diagnosis and management of stroke (publication is expected
for 2008).

heparin was compared with a no-heparin control group (2% versus 5%; p=0.001) (1+). However, the trial also found that the incidence of haemorrhagic stroke was higher in the heparin group (2.8% versus 0.4%), thus offsetting the reduction in ischaemic stroke. (1+)

No significant association has been found between the use of aspirin in comparison with either placebo or control and the incidence of acute recurrent stroke (ischaemic or haemorrhagic) or acute mortality (2 to 4 weeks post-stroke).[260] (1+)

11.2.3 From evidence to recommendations

It was agreed that there were little data on which to formulate an evidence-based recommendation on when to initiate oral anticoagulation in a patient with AF following a stroke or TIA. In the absence of evidence, it was therefore agreed to base recommendations on pre-existing guidelines in the area.[202]

It was agreed that cerebral imaging may be performed (by MRI or CT scan) to exclude haemorrhage, and antithrombotic therapy should commence at approximatey 2 weeks after the stroke or TIA where there is no evidence of haemorrhage. It should be noted, however, that the discrimination between haemorrhage and ischaemic stroke with CT scanning can only be made reliably within a few days of the event. At later times gradient echo MRI may be the only reliable method.

In patients with AF who have had a large infarction or uncontrolled hypertension, antithrombotic therapy may be delayed. Although AF is widely recognised as a significant risk factor for ischaemic stroke, patients with AF may have other risk factors. AF may not be responsible for all strokes occurring in AF patients. Nonetheless, secondary stroke prevention is warranted and AF patients who have experienced an ischaemic stroke will benefit from appropriate antithrombotic therapy according to the recommendations below and the stroke risk stratification algorithm (Figure 11.1) regardless of aetiology.

RECOMMENDATIONS

R49   In all patients with AF who have had an acute stroke, any uncontrolled hypertension
       should be appropriately managed before antithrombotic therapy is started.   D(GPP)

R50   In patients with AF and an acute stroke:
       • imaging (CT scan or MRI) should be performed to exclude cerebral haemorrhage
       • in the absence of haemorrhage, anticoagulation therapy should begin after 2 weeks
       • in the presence of haemorrhage, anticoagulation therapy should not be given
       • in the presence of a large cerebral infarction, the initiation of anticoagulation
         therapy should be delayed.   D(GPP)

R51   In patients with AF and an acute TIA:
       • imaging (CT scan or MRI) should be performed to exclude recent cerebral infarction or
         haemorrhage
       • in the absence of cerebral infarction or haemorrhage, anticoagulation therapy
         should begin as soon as possible.   D(GPP)

11.3 Antithrombotic therapy following a stroke or TIA

AF is an independent predictor of stroke[13] with the risk approximately five times that of people without AF. The absolute risk for an individual patient, however, increases with age and depends upon the presence of other risk factors such as valvular heart disease, other cardiovascular disease or cardiac risk factors. Conversely, anticoagulation therapy substantially reduces the risk of stroke in 'at risk' patients with AF.[174,260]

In stroke patients, concurrent AF is associated with greater disability, longer in-hospital patient stay and lower rate of discharge to their own home, and in most studies AF is associated with decreased survival.[261,262]

Patients who have suffered and survived an acute stroke or transient ischaemic attack are at the highest risk of recurrent stroke and thromboembolism, approximately 12% per year.[258] Assessment and treatment of comorbidities (especially hypertension) is essential, as is an accurate risk–benefit assessment. The highest risk patients are the elderly, and this is probably the group where anticoagulation treatment is most difficult.

The objective of this section is to provide evidence-based guidelines on which is the best thromboprophylactic agent for post-stroke AF patients.

11.3.1 Methodological introduction

Five primary studies[258,259,263–265] and two meta-analyses[266,267] were identified. One study[258] was included in both meta-analyses. One study compared warfarin, aspirin and placebo.[258] All studies recruited AF patients with a prior stroke or TIA except one[179] that included 44% of AF patients without a prior stroke or TIA.

11.3.2 Evidence statements

One meta-analysis[266] found warfarin to be associated with a reduced incidence of recurrent stroke (ischaemic or haemorrhagic) and vascular events (including stroke, myocardial infarction, systemic embolism and vascular death) but an increased incidence of bleeding events, compared with placebo. (1+)

There was no significant difference in the mortality rate between adjusted-dose warfarin and placebo.[258] (1++)

Low molecular weight heparin is associated with a significant reduction in embolic events and overall mortality when compared with no treatment.[265] (1+)

Acenocoumarol administered to a target INR of 1.25 to 2.00, in conjunction with 600mg/day triflusal, reduces the incidence of stroke (ischaemic or haemorrhagic), vascular death or systemic embolism compared with acenocoumarol alone administered to a target INR of 2.0 to 3.0179 (1+). No association has been found in rates of severe bleeding or overall incidence of adverse events.[179] (1+)

Adjusted dose warfarin is associated with a reduced incidence of recurrent stroke (ischaemic or haemorrhagic),[258,264] and vascular events[258] compared with aspirin (1++). Warfarin has also been found to be associated with an increased incidence of bleeding events compared with aspirin.[258] (1++)

No significant difference has been found in the mortality rate between adjusted-dose warfarin and aspirin.[258] (1++)

Warfarin has been found to be associated with a greater reduction in the incidence of overall stroke recurrence following a presumed primary cardioembolic stroke in comparison with aspirin, but not following a presumed primary lacunar stroke.[258] (1++)

No significant difference between aspirin and placebo has been found in the overall incidence of vascular events, mortality or bleeding events.[258] (1++)

No association has been found between the use of dipyridamole and placebo in the incidence of recurrent ischaemic stroke. A similar result was found when dipyridamole was combined with aspirin and compared with placebo.[264] (1++)

11.3.3 From evidence to recommendations

Anticoagulation with warfarin has a strong beneficial effect in the prevention of recurrent strokes for post-stroke and post-TIA patients with AF when compared with both placebo[258,266] and aspirin.[267] This effect is significant for any category of secondary stroke. However, anticoagulation also increases rates of haemorrhagic events in comparison with both placebo and aspirin.

The GDG agreed that antiplatelet agents such as aspirin and dipyridamole are ineffective thromboprophylactic agents and should be administered to post-stroke AF patients only to treat other comorbidities or vascular disease.

The GDG noted that the use of low adjusted-dose anticoagulation with acenocoumarol in combination with the antiplatelet triflusal was more effective than conventional adjusted-dose anticoagulation with acenocoumarol alone for the prevention of stroke.[179] It is unclear whether similar results apply to anticoagulation with warfarin instead of acenocoumarol or other antiplatelet agents. The GDG noted that trifusal is not used in the UK, and that previous studies of warfarin and aspirin combination therapy have been less effective or have had more adverse effects than with warfarin alone. Therefore the GDG did not make any recommendations in this area.

RECOMMENDATIONS

R52 In patients with AF who are either post-stroke, or have had a TIA:
* warfarin should be administered as the most effective thromboprophylactic agent   A
* aspirin or dipyridamole should not be administered as thromboprophylactic agents unless indicated for the treatment of comorbidities or vascular disease.   D(GPP)

R53 Treatment of post-stroke or post-TIA patients with warfarin should only begin after treatment of relevant comorbidities (such as hypertension) and assessment of the risk–benefit ratio.   D(GPP)

11.4 Antithrombotic therapy for asymptomatic AF

Many patients develop AF asymptomatically, and only present to medical care when complications such as stroke or heart failure occur. One study reported that in patients with paroxysmal AF, only 1 in 12 paroxysms appeared to be symptomatic.[31] Consequently, cases of AF are often detected, particularly in the elderly, during a general practice visit for an unrelated problem. The elderly, as a group, have a high morbidity from stroke, thromboembolism and impaired cognitive function.

It is not known whether asymptomatic AF *per se* is a potential risk factor for stroke. It is currently not clear how best to manage patients with asymptomatic AF, either in relation to treatment using a rate-control or a rhythm-control strategy, or in terms of the need for antithrombotic therapy.

11.4.1 Methodological introduction

No studies were found that addressed this clinical area.

11.4.2 From evidence to recommendations

The GDG noted that there was no evidence upon which to base recommendations on the use of antithrombotic therapy in patients with asymptomatic AF. The group noted that many patients had AF diagnosed but that the opportunity for antithrombotic therapy was not always considered. The group agreed that asymptomatic AF should be treated no differently to symptomatic AF.

RECOMMENDATION

R54   Patients with asymptomatic AF should receive thromboprophylaxis as for symptomatic
AF (refer to section 6.3 for persistent AF, section 7.2 for permanent AF and section 8.2
for paroxysmal AF).   D(GPP)

11.5 Risks of long-term anticoagulation

In order to provide adequate thromboprophylaxis with minimal risk of bleeding, current clinical practice aims for a target INR of between 2.0 and 3.0; INRs of more than 3.0 are associated with increases in bleeding and INRs of less than 2.0 are associated with increases in stroke risk.[176,182]

In one pooled analysis, the annual rate of major haemorrhage (defined as an intracranial haemorrhage, a haemorrhage requiring at least two units of blood, or an event requiring hospital admission) was 1% in control patients and 1.3% in warfarin-treated patients.[168] The annual risks of intracranial haemorrhage increased from 0.1% in control to 0.3% in warfarin groups, which represents an excess of two intracranial bleeds per annum per 1,000 patients treated. Even low-dose aspirin increases the risk of major haemorrhage by two-fold, especially in the settling of uncontrolled hypertension. Indeed, the correct treatment and monitoring of hypertension and other associated comorbidities is regarded as extremely important in minimising the risk of bleeding in patients on prophylactic warfarin.

The most devastating complication associated with warfarin prophylaxis is the risk of intracranial haemorrhage, which is a particular problem in the elderly, in whom frailty, poor mobility, forgetfulness or poor compliance with medication, concomitant medications (resulting in drug interactions), and frequent falls may jeopardise the benefits from warfarin. These factors are often cited as reasons for non-prescription of warfarin in the elderly, where the absolute benefit is likely to be greatest in view of their high risk.[169]

There is also some evidence[268] that the combined use of warfarin with antiplatelet agents such as aspirin and clopidogrel significantly increases the risk of bleeding beyond that associated with the single use of any one of these agents. This raises a particular dilemma in those patients with both atrial fibrillation and coronary or peripheral artery disease, who are often co-prescribed warfarin and antiplatelet therapy. With the increasing use of drug-eluting stents, for which 6 to 12 months aspirin-clopidogrel use has recently been recommended, advice on how best to manage patients who have both AF and a drug-eluting stent who also require anticoagulation is currently lacking.[269]

This section aims to identify those risk factors for bleeding in patients with AF receiving oral anticoagulation.

11.5.1 Methodological introduction

'Long-term' anticoagulation was assumed to mean periods of anticoagulation administration of longer than 4 weeks. Studies that considered outcomes in populations with a mean period of anticoagulation of less than 4 weeks were excluded.

Studies were included in this report if they documented the incidence of complications associated with long-term oral anticoagulation, such as drug toxicity or adverse side effects, and measured and compared the risk of these complications between different groups of patients.

The reporting of risk will be made for both multivariate risk analyses, as well as univariate associations, wherever a multivariate calculation has not been reported.

11.5.2 Evidence statements

▷ Overall bleeding risk

One large study[270] (N=10,093) in an elderly population (mean age 77 years), reported a yearly incidence of 1.5% major bleeding events, of which 0.3% were intracranial haemorrhage.[28]

In another study[271] (N=677), in a population receiving both anticoagulation and antiplatelet therapy, the yearly incidence of major bleeding events was 1.1%, of which 0.6% were intracranial haemorrhage.[28] The study reported a yearly incidence of 11.8% minor bleeding events.[28]

▷ Bleeding risk factors

One study[272] found that patients older than 75 years were more likely to suffer bleeding complications than younger patients (2+). A similar result was found in another study.[273] (2+)

One small study[274] (N=101) did not find any significant difference in the incidence of bleeding complications between those aged 75 years or over and those aged 60 to 69 years. (2+)

Four studies[270,272,275,276] found no association between gender and bleeding complications, although female gender was found to be of borderline significance as an independent risk factor in two other studies.[270] (2+)

One study[271] failed to find diabetes to be a significant independent risk factor of bleeding complications (2+). A further three studies[272,275,276] failed to find any significant association between diabetes and bleeding. (2+)

One study[271] did not find hypertension to be a significant predictor of bleeding complications, although another larger study[168] found both systolic and diastolic blood pressure to be significantly higher in those patients with bleeding complications than in those without bleeding complications. (2+)

One study[270] found anaemia to be significantly associated with bleeding complications in an elderly cohort of patients. (2+)

Two studies[271,276] found a history of MI to be a significant independent predictor of bleeding complications (2+). A similar result was found for the presence of ischaemic heart disease.[276] (2+)

Two studies[271,272] failed to find a history of stroke or thromboembolism to be independent predictors of bleeding complications. (2+)

One study[276] did not find any significant association between cerebrovascular disease and incidence of bleeding complications although another larger study[277] found cerebrovascular disease to be a significant independent predictor of intracranial haemorrhage. (2++)

One study[270] found the concomitant use of antiplatelet drugs in anticoagulated patients to be a significant independent predictor of bleeding complications (2+). However, the same study did not find an increased number of additional medications – including non-steroidal anti-inflammatory drugs (NSAIDs) – to be a significant independent predictor of bleeding complications when risk was correlated with an increase of one additional drug. (2+)

One study[278] found a significant difference in bleeding complications between those patients prescribed at least three additional medications and those prescribed less than three. (2++)

One study[270] found a history of bleeding to be a significant independent predictor of future bleeding events. (2+)

11.5.3 From evidence to recommendations

The following risk factors were identified as being associated with bleeding in AF cohorts:

- over 75 years of age
- antiplatelet drug use
- uncontrolled hypertension
- history of bleeding or ICH
- anaemia
- polypharmacy.

It was considered unclear whether controlled hypertension or previous MI were independent predictors of stroke. For example, patients with previous MI were likely to be taking antiplatelet therapy, and may have other comorbidities, such as uncontrolled hypertension. Anaemia was a risk factor in the studies presented, probably because of an underlying bleeding source (eg peptic ulcer).

Poor anticoagulation control could also be considered as another risk factor for bleeding, particularly since the risk increased with INRs of greater than 3.0.[277] The use of concomitant antiplatelet therapy (aspirin or clopidogrel) was identified as a risk factor to bleeding; NSAIDs were thought to have a similar risk. Obvious bleeding factors, such as recent bleeding peptic ulcer or intracranial bleeding, are contraindications to anticoagulation, in view of the high risk associated with these conditions.

One criticism of the randomised trials is that they do not reflect real world practice, only randomising a minority of those screened, who tended to be at lower risk and monitored closely by intense trial protocols. One prospective UK cohort study, designed to determine if trial efficacy of warfarin for stroke prevention in AF translated into clinical effectiveness, reported that the rate of stroke (2% per year, 95% CI 0.7 to 4.4) compared with patients in the pooled studies (1.4% per year). Major bleeding rates (1.7% versus 1.6%) were also comparable.[176,279,280]

It was noted that many of the risk factors for bleeding (eg aged over 75 years, hypertension) were also risk factors for stroke (see section 11.6). Thus, it may be appropriate to undertake an assessment of bleeding risk as part of the clinical assessment of patients prior to starting antithrombotic therapy.

RECOMMENDATIONS

R55   Both the antithrombotic benefits and the potential bleeding risks of long-term anticoagulation should be explained to and discussed with the patient.   D(GPP)

R56   The assessment of bleeding risk should be part of the clinical assessment of patients before starting anticoagulation therapy. Particular attention should be paid to patients who:

- are over 75 years of age   D
- are taking antiplatelet drugs (such as aspirin or clopidogrel) or non-steroidal anti-inflammatory drugs   C
- are on multiple other drug treatments (polypharmacy)   C
- have uncontrolled hypertension   C
- have a history of bleeding (for example, peptic ulcer or cerebral haemorrhage)   C
- have a history of poorly controlled anticoagulation therapy.   D(GPP)

11.6 Risk factors for stroke and thromboembolism

AF itself is an independent risk factor for stroke[14] and results in an independent increase in mortality *per se.*[11]

Stroke risk is also perceived to vary according to age and the presence of hypertension, diabetes mellitus, previous stroke or transient ischemic attack and poor cardiac function.

Transthoracic and transoesophageal echocardiography features have also been associated with a high risk of stroke (see section 4.3). Echocardiography therefore complements risk stratification on clinical grounds.

The objective of this section is to identify those risk factors for stroke or thromboembolism in patients with AF that should be incorporated into a comprehensive risk stratification algorithm.

11.6.1 Methodological introduction

All of the included studies were based in populations where the vast majority of people were receiving no anticoagulant drug during the course of the study period, and which identified independent risk factors of stroke or thromboembolism.

The use of aspirin or any other drug with presumed antithrombotic efficacy will not be reported here as a (negative) risk factor for stroke or thromboembolism. Echocardiographic risk factors are considered elsewhere (see section 4.3).

Although many studies considered the composite outcome of (ischaemic) stroke, TIA or thromboembolism, for the purposes of brevity this report will refer to the entire range of outcomes simply as 'stroke'.

11.6.2 Evidence statements

▷ Demographic risk factors

Of 10 studies that considered increasing age as a risk factor for stroke, either as a continuous variable or as incremental decades, six[168,192,281–284] found increasing age to be a significant risk factor, while the remaining studies[59,285–287] did not find increasing age to be significant. (2++)

Of three studies[60,288,289] that considered being elderly as a risk factor for stroke (by dichotomising age into younger and older age groups), one relatively small (N=272) study[60] did not find being aged over 70 years to be a significant risk factor (2+). In another study[288] (N=740) in a population with intermittent AF (at enrolment), being aged over 65 years was a significant risk factor for stroke (RR 3.3, 95% CI 1.92 to 5.81) (2+). In another study[289] (N=265) of a population without a previous stroke, being aged over 75 years was a significant risk factor for stroke (OR 1.72, 95% CI 1.04 to 2.84). (2+)

Based on the results of 11 studies[52,59,60,62,192,281–283,285,286,288] in various populations of AF patients, it is unclear whether gender is a significant independent risk factor. (2++)

One study[290] (N=854) found being female and over 75 years old to be a significant independent predictor of stroke (OR 3.7, 95% CI 2.2 to 6.2; p<0.001). (2++)

One study[168] (N=1593) did not find smoking to be a significant independent predictor of stroke (2+). However, the study did find a higher incidence of stroke in smokers than non-smokers (p<0.05). (2+)

▷ Clinical risk factors

Seven studies[62,168,192,281,283,284,287] found a history of stroke or TIA to be a significant independent predictor of secondary stroke (2++). Another study[285] based in a population with a prior stroke or TIA found a previous non-cerebrovascular thromboembolism to be a significant independent predictor of secondary stroke. (2++)

Based on the results of seven studies,[52,168,192,281,282,289,291] hypertension (controlled or uncontrolled) has been found to be a significant independent risk factor in both AF and atrial flutter (2++). However, another four studies[60,62,284,286] failed to find any significant relationship between hypertension and stroke. (2++)

Three studies[192,281,285] found systolic blood pressure greater than 160 mm Hg to be a significant independent predictor of stroke in general AF populations (2++). However, one study[192] failed to find it to be a significant independent risk factor specifically in patients with intermittent AF. (1+)

Based on the results of eight studies[52,60,62,168,282,284,287,290] that considered various measures of structural heart disease as risk factors for stroke, it is unclear whether congestive heart failure (CHF) is a risk factor for stroke[168,282,284,287] (2++), although the presence of structural heart disease generally has been found to be a significant independent predictor.[60] (2+)

One study[282] did not find the presence of ischaemic heart disease to be a significant independent predictor of stroke (2++). A similar result was found in the case of angina in another study.[168] (2+)

Two studies[168] found the presence of diabetes to be a significant independent predictor of stroke in a general AF population (2+). Another study[62] based in an elderly population did not find it to be an independent risk factor. (2+)

Two studies[282,286] based in AF populations without a previous stroke[286] or without any risk factors, including previous stroke and presence of CHF or left ventricular dysfunction,[282] did not find diabetes to be a significant independent predictor of stroke (2++). One study[291] based in a population with atrial flutter did not find diabetes to be a significant independent predictor of stroke. (2+)

Four studies considered a history of MI as a risk factor for stroke. Three studies[52,168,286] found MI to a significant independent risk factor (2+). The remaining study[62] based in an elderly population did not find MI to be a significant independent risk factor. (2+)

Two studies[60,284] did not find AF subtype (paroxysmal or non-paroxysmal) to be a significant independent predictor of stroke. (2++)

One study[285] based in a population with a previous stroke or TIA found an AF duration of greater than 1 year to be a significant independent predictor of secondary stroke. (2++)

One study[62] did not find obesity to be a significant independent predictor of stroke. (2+)

11.6.3 From evidence to recommendations

Many of the studies used highly selected populations that would affect the relative risk of the factors considered. The main data appraised came from cohort studies, epidemiological studies and clinical trials. Many of the clinical trials randomised only a small proportion of those initially screened, and excluded patients with valvular heart disease, thyroid disease or intercurrent illnesses such as chest infections.

Based on the evidence, the following were identified as independent risk factors for stroke in AF:
- previous stroke or TIA
- being elderly (aged over 75)
- structural heart disease
- hypertension
- previous MI.

The evidence for diabetes as an independent predictor of stroke in AF was not considered convincing, but overall was regarded as an important indicator for increased risk in the general AF population.

While MI was identified as an independent stroke risk factor, underlying left ventricular dysfunction may confound this result. Echocardiographically demonstrated left ventricular dysfunction is a known risk factor for stroke, but heart failure cannot always be diagnosed on clinical grounds alone. It was therefore agreed that heart failure should be on the list of risk factors even though the evidence was inconclusive.

Other risk factors such as peripheral artery disease were debated, but limited evidence was available. However, coronary and peripheral artery diseases were regarded as part of the clinical spectrum of atherothrombotic vascular disease that contributed to stroke risk. For example, complex aortic plaque on TOE was an independent stroke risk factor[292] (see section 4.3) and ischaemic stroke in AF could be associated with carotid artery disease.[293] For this reason vascular disease should be incorporated into a risk stratification model.

The evidence was unclear as to whether being female is a stroke risk factor. It was agreed that there was no known plausible biological reason for females with AF to have a higher stroke risk than men, and it was thus agreed that being female should not be included in any risk stratification algorithm.

Although none of the appraised studies considered AF patients with thyroid disease, it was agreed that this should not be considered as a risk factor for stroke.

All of the above factors, which are not mutually exclusive and may be cumulative, have been used in the development of various risk stratification algorithms (see Appendix B). These algorithms have been designed to assist the clinician in assessing individual patients for thromboprophylaxis. They can help in the identification of patients with AF who are at an increased risk of stroke and who would benefit most from anticoagulation therapy, while low-risk patients could be managed with antiplatelet therapy.

There is a need for an algorithm that stratifies stroke risk into three tiers to allow:
- high-risk patients to be identified for thromboprophylaxic anticoagulation therapy
- low-risk patients to be identified for antiplatelet use for thromboprophylaxis
- moderate-risk patients to be identified where further specialist referral may be necessary.

In addition to risk stratification it was accepted that patients preferences should be considered as some patients will still decline anticoagulation treatment for a variety of reasons. These include:

- the inconvenience of dosing adjustments and regular blood tests to monitor INR levels
- dietary restrictions
- the risk of minor and major bleeding, and
- under-appreciation or lack of knowledge regarding the risk of stroke, or poor adherence to the treatment regimen.

Many patients with AF possess limited knowledge of AF and its consequences and therapy. Only a minority reported feeling that their doctor had given them enough information about their warfarin therapy.

The following criteria were identified that should be addressed by any risk stratification algorithm for use in a UK population:

- incorporation of the risk factors identified above
- inclusion of a three-strata model (high, moderate and low risk)
- easy to use (no complex scoring system)
- patients with previous stroke or TIA automatically classified as high risk
- can be used for both primary and secondary prevention
- practical and applicable for use in both primary and secondary care.

A summary of the published risk stratification algorithms is shown in Appendix B. The benefits and drawbacks of each were discussed, with emphasis on a balance between evidence, clinical applicability and practicality, as well as refinement for a UK population. It was agreed that few had addressed the cumulative nature of risk factors where a combination (eg hypertension plus diabetes) would confer a greater risk than either alone.

It was noted that none of the published algorithms had been derived or validated in a UK population but one had subsequently been modified for this purpose.[294] Various other problems were highlighted regarding the applicability of the published algorithms:

- With the exception of one model,[283] non-warfarin trial participants had often been used as validation populations.
- One was based on a complex mathematical model.[283]
- Some only used a two-tier model (low and moderate–high risk) to stratify patients.[28,168,290,295]
- One was based on a point scoring system.[296]
- One did not necessarily identify a patient with a previous stroke or TIA as 'high risk'.[296]
- One model was only applicable for secondary prevention.[285]

It was agreed to suggest a revised algorithm based on the only model that had been optimised for use in a UK setting.[294] This was based on a modification of the AF investigators' algorithm,[168] but had been expanded into a three-tier model following consultation with primary and secondary care clinicians and was implemented (31/08/1997) and subsequently validated as a regional audit project in primary care by a large UK health authority.

RECOMMENDATIONS

R57   The stroke risk stratification algorithm (section 11.7) should be used in patients with AF to assess their risk of stroke and thromboembolism, and appropriate thromboprophylaxis given.   C

R58   Risk stratification should be reconsidered whenever individual risk factors are reviewed.   D(GPP)

11.7 Stroke risk stratification algorithm

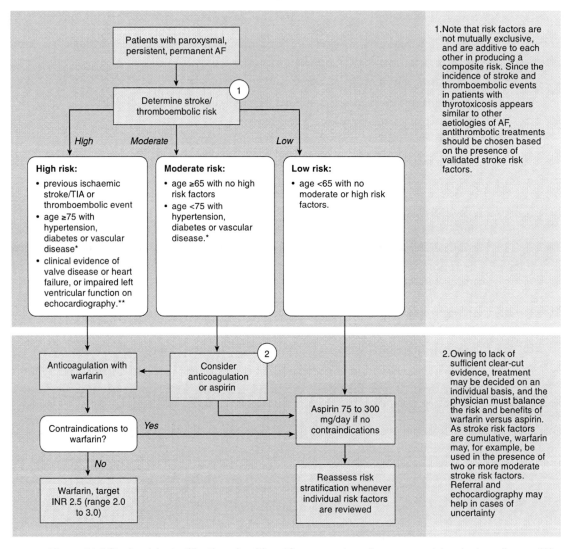

Figure 11.1 Stroke risk stratification algorithm. *Coronary artery disease or peripheral artery disease. **An echocardiogram is not needed for routine assessment, but refines clinical risk stratification in the case of moderate or severe LV dysfunction and valve disease.

11.8 The cost effectiveness of oral anticoagulation as thromboprophylaxis

The purpose of this section is to consider the health economic aspects of oral anticoagulation in patients with AF. In particular, since the risk of stroke is not homogenous throughout the AF population (see section 11.6), the administration of oral anticoagulation as thrombo-prophylaxis may be cost effective in high-risk patients, but not cost effective in lower risk patients. In those patients in whom oral anticoagulation is not cost effective, antiplatelet therapy may be more appropriate, or no treatment.

11.8.1 Methodological introduction

Eight published cost-effectiveness studies compared warfarin with no anticoagulation and/or warfarin with aspirin. Five of the cost-effectiveness studies were US-based,[297–301] two were conducted in the UK[302,303] and one in Sweden.[304]

Discounted survival or quality-adjusted survival was estimated using the prevalence over time of stroke, haemorrhagic events and mortality associated with AF. The ranges of outcomes incorporated in the models were very similar. All the studies drew from a relatively robust, up-to-date evidence of effectiveness of warfarin in preventing strokes. This is also presented in the review of effectiveness and consists of a meta-analysis of the effectiveness of warfarin in non-valvular AF patients.[305]

Most studies considered a healthcare system perspective (NHS for the two UK studies) and included discounted, direct costs of anticoagulation therapy (physicians or outpatient visits, drugs and prescription costs) and costs of hospitalisation for stroke and major haemorrhagic events.

11.8.2 Evidence statements

▷ Anticoagulation versus no anticoagulation

In general patients with AF, anticoagulation treatment is relatively cost effective compared with no anticoagulation. Three studies[297,300,302] reported on cost effectiveness of warfarin compared with no warfarin in a general AF population. The only UK study[302] reported an ICER ranging between £1,751 and £13,221 per life-year gained free from stroke. Studies from other countries reported cost-effectiveness ratios of US$1,907.[297] Another study[304] estimated that the cost per stroke prevented stratified according to risk of bleeding to be Swedish krona (SKR)171,000 per stroke prevented if the risk of bleeding is 0.3%, to SKR417,000 if the risk of bleeding is 2%. The other study[300] estimated a reduction in healthcare costs of US$1,514 per year.

Four studies[297–299,303] compared anticoagulation with no anticoagulation in patients with a low risk of stroke. In this subgroup of patients anticoagulation was found not to be cost effective, with higher costs and loss in quality of life compared with no anticoagulation.

In patients with medium to high risk for stroke, anticoagulation with warfarin was found to be cost effective, with estimated ICERs ranging between dominance[297,298] and ICERs of between US$1,434/QALY[299] and £6,000/QALY.[303] One study[303] also found that the ICER decreased as blood pressure increased.

In patients at high risk of stroke (more than two risk factors of stroke) all studies[297–299,303] found that anticoagulation was dominant, ie had lower costs and improved quality adjusted survival.

In elderly patients, the cost effectiveness of anticoagulation was found to depend on the level of risk of stroke. For high-risk patients, the ICERs ranged between dominance (lower costs and better outcomes) for individuals with high-risk factors.[297,299,302] For low-risk patients, anticoagulation was dominated by no anticoagulation.

▷ Anticoagulation versus antiplatelet therapy

Three studies[297,300,302] compared anticoagulation treatment with aspirin in general patients with AF. The ICERs ranged from US$2,000 in patients with low implantable cardiac defibrillator (ICH) risk (0.2%) to approximately US$7,000 in patients with high ICH risk (1.2%).[380] One study[297] had an ICER of US$4484/quality-adjusted life-years (QALY) while another study[300] found that warfarin treatment resulted in cost savings. Thus, in general patients with AF, warfarin was found to be cost effective compared with aspirin.

In low-risk patients, one study[298] estimated small improvements in QALYs which were realised at substantial costs compared with aspirin (US$370,000/QALY for 65 year olds and US$110,000/QALY for 75-year-olds).

In patients with AF who have a medium to high risk of stroke, one study[298] calculated an ICER of US$8,000/QALY for anticoagulation with warfarin. The cost-effectiveness advantage was found to decrease as the risk of bleeding increased.

In elderly patients with a moderate risk of stroke, one study[298] found that warfarin was cost effective compared with aspirin with an estimated ICER of US$500/QALY.

11.8.3 Evidence to recommendations

The health economic analysis suggested that the studies comparing warfarin with no anticoagulation and warfarin with aspirin were of good quality and summarised the evidence as follows:

- In patients with AF, anticoagulation treatment is cost effective compared with no anticoagulation.
- In patients at high risk of stroke, anticoagulation is cost effective, but not for those with a low risk of stroke.
- Aspirin is cost effective in low-risk patients compared with warfarin, but not in higher risk patients.

It was agreed that the health economics evidence was consistent with the stroke risk stratification algorithm (Figure 11.1).

12 | Monitoring and referral

12.1 Anticoagulation self-monitoring

The increasing use of oral anticoagulation therapy as thromboprophylaxis in AF has increased the need for anticoagulation monitoring and encouraged a move towards 'point of care' or 'near patient' testing and patient self-monitoring. This may take several forms, whereby the patient has an anticoagulation-monitoring test performed at:

- the GP clinic using an INR testing machine based in the clinic itself, or
- the GP clinic but using an INR testing machine based in a central laboratory (normally at a hospital) where the blood sample is sent, or
- home using a personal INR testing machine allowing the patient to alter the dose of anticoagulation (self-monitoring).

Point of care for INR testing within primary care eliminates time lost in waiting for test results to be processed, by informing the patient of any changes to their INR and of any resulting change in dosing advice.[306]

Patient self-monitoring of oral anticoagulation gives a greater degree of autonomy. However, evidence is also required regarding the clinical utility and cost effectiveness of self-monitoring in order to recommend its routine use in clinical practice.

This section provides an opportunity to assess the evidence on whether self-monitoring is as effective as management using hospital laboratory testing and other conventional management strategies.

12.1.1 Methodological introduction

Studies were included if self-monitoring strategies were compared with traditional supervised-management strategies for the monitoring and dose-adjustment of long-term oral anti-coagulation. In the former case, self-monitoring could involve either the patient testing their own INR values and recording those values for appraisal by a supervising clinician responsible for dose-adjustment, or the patient performing both their own INR testing and dose-adjustment. In the latter case, testing was performed centrally or by clinicians using near-patient testing devices and clinicians made the dose-adjustment decisions.

The manufacturer or local distributor of the testing device funded all of the studies, either directly or indirectly.

Two studies had populations solely comprising AF patients.[307,308] The other studies included a proportion of AF patients within a general anticoagulated population[309-316] and others either included only patients with prosthetic heart valves[317,318] or did not report the number of patients with AF.[319-321] However, the results of the studies were consistent across all patient populations. A recently published meta-analysis[322] of 10 of the RCTs included in the guideline review was subsequently identified. The pooled results for relevant outcomes are included in the evidence statements below.

Two studies[323,324] were found that reported health economic outcomes of self-monitoring in comparison with supervised management. One study[323] was a cost-effectiveness analysis and the other[324] developed a comparative cost analysis where cost functions were developed and analysed to determine the break-even point in total cost between the two systems.

12.1.2 Evidence statements

Based on the results of 10 studies,[307,308,311,314–7,319–21] it is inconclusive whether self-monitoring is associated with improved control of INR compared with supervised management, when measured as the percentage of INR measurements within the target range. (1++)

No difference was found in the number of dose adjustments per INR measurement between self-monitoring (0.42) and supervised management (0.37)[312] (2++). However, the number of dose adjustments per patient was higher in the self-monitoring group (22.4 versus 3.4; $p<0.005$).[312] (2++)

Self-monitoring is associated with a lower rate of hospital admissions than supervised management in patients with prosthetic heart valves (15.3% versus 9.5%; $p<0.05$).[311] (1+)

When comparing self-management and supervised-management strategies, no significant association was found within individual studies in the rates of major thromboembolic or haemorrhagic complications.[307,310,312–315,318–20] A meta-analysis[322] of eight RCTs found self-management to be associated with significantly fewer major thromboembolic events (OR 0.41, 95% CI 0.25 to 0.70; $p=0.001$), but failed to detect a significant association for haemorrhagic complications (OR 0.66, 95% CI 0.37 to 1.16; $p=0.15$). (1++)

No significant difference in mortality rates between self-management and supervised-management strategies was detected within individual studies.[307,312,313,315,317–319] A meta-analysis[322] of five RCTs found self-management to be associated with significantly fewer deaths from all causes (OR 0.58, 95% CI 0.36 to 0.95; $p=0.03$). (1++)

One study[321] reported a higher incidence of major complications in those patients with conventional management than those with self-monitoring (7.3% versus 2.2%). (1+)

Self-monitoring was associated with a higher level of patient satisfaction and quality of life than supervised management when assessed by questionnaires.[313,318] (1++)

One cohort study reported patient preferences after study termination and 15 of the 17 patients from the self-monitoring group bought a near-patient testing device[307] (2++). The remaining two participants expressed a wish to purchase one but were financially unable to do so.

No significant association has been found between self-monitoring strategies that allow dose adjustment by patients and those where dose adjustment was determined by a clinician in terms of either the percentage of time spent within the target INR range (67% self-testing only versus 69% self-testing and self-dosing) or the percentage of measurements within the target INR range (64% self-testing only versus 66% self-testing and self-dosing).[314] (1++)

The cost-effectiveness results differed depending on whether or not costs incurred by patients and their carers are included with medical care costs.[323] Anticoagulation clinic testing versus usual care was cost saving when including medical costs only (US$405,560 versus US$419,514). Patient self-testing versus anticoagulation clinic testing had an incremental cost of US$24,818 per adverse event avoided or US$153,504 per QALY when including medical costs only. However, when including all costs, patient self-testing versus anticoagulation clinic testing was cost saving (US$622,727 versus US$645,671). Patient self-testing had higher medical care costs than usual care (US$526,014 versus US$419,514) but had a lower number of adverse events per 100 patients over 5 years (22.10 versus 30.65).

Results were sensitive to time spent below or above the therapeutic INR range and frequency of testing. Including medical costs only, there is approximately 80% certainty that anticoagulation clinic testing versus usual care is cost saving, and 48% certainty that patient self-testing versus anticoagulation clinic testing is cost saving.[323]

The use of near-patient testing costs less per year than conventional anticoagulation follow-up in self-care patients (€350.37N versus €378.36N, where N=number of patients). The yearly cost of near-patient testing is €133.77 plus €953.02N and equals the cost of conventional follow-up (€963.00N) when there are more than 14 patients on home-care follow-up. Sensitivity analysis indicates that small changes in the cost of near-patient management could affect the number of patients needed to make the near-patient model cost effective. The results were also sensitive to the travel costs.[324]

12.1.3 From evidence to recommendations

The evidence suggests that patient self-monitoring of oral anticoagulation is more effective in terms of patient satisfaction than supervised management.[313] However, the results of such trials should be interpreted carefully.

Many studies were conducted using a motivated patient population who were selected using strict inclusion criteria, which often included passing a cognitive test. In one study[307] the authors report that although at the end of the study period many patients wished to continue self-monitoring, this required sufficient personal financial resource to fund the purchase of the necessary equipment.

There was a difference in the cost effectiveness depending on whether patient and carer costs were included with medical costs. Further data based on the UK health setting would be required in order to determine the cost effectiveness of self-monitoring.

A recent non-commercially funded trial[325] which was published too late to be included in the above review, showed self-monitoring to be safe and effective in a UK population. This conclusion is consistent with the results from smaller trials above, most of which received commercial backing.

Increasing the adoption of self-monitoring might lead to additional pressure on GP services. It was considered that the use of self-monitoring needs to be balanced between patient preference and the ability of local services to provide support (eg patient education programmes).

It was noted that guidelines have been published in the area of patient self-monitoring of oral anticoagulation.[326] These recommend that patients undertaking anticoagulation self-monitoring should be trained by a competent healthcare professional and remain in contact with a named clinician. They also highlight the need for self-monitoring devices that have been adequately quality-assured.

RECOMMENDATION

R59   In patients with AF who require long-term anticoagulation, self-monitoring should be considered if preferred by the patient and the following criteria are met:

- the patient is both physically and cognitively able to perform the self-monitoring test, or in those cases where the patient is not physically or cognitively able to perform self-monitoring, a designated carer is able to do so
- an adequate supportive educational programme is in place to train patients and/or carers
- the patient's ability to self-manage is regularly reviewed
- the equipment for self-monitoring is regularly checked via a quality control programme.   C

12.2 Follow-up post cardioversion

In current clinical practice review of patients after successful cardioversion is primarily to assess the maintenance of sinus rhythm. In addition the following factors are also considered:

- comorbid factors (eg heart failure, hypertension), by review
- adverse effects related to cardioversion (eg skin burns, thromboembolism)
- drug therapies (eg proarrhythmia from antiarrhythmic drugs, or bleeding from anticoagulation), and
- likelihood of arrhythmia recurrence, by assessment.

Those patients considered most likely to successfully cardiovert and maintain sinus rhythm are those who have recent onset AF (less than 12 months), those with no underlying structural heart disease, and those who have AF secondary to a precipitant (eg treated thyroid disease, fever) that has been successfully treated or corrected.

The consideration of symptoms alone as indicators of AF recurrence is not usually reliable, since many instances of recurrence occur asymptomatically.[64]

For patients with AF recurrence the decision needs to be made of whether another attempt at cardioversion should be undertaken, or a strategy of rate control should be adopted (see section 6.3), and whether the patient requires long-term antithrombotic therapy (see section 11.6).

12.2.1 Methodological introduction

Fifteen studies were included that compared different electrophysiological, radiological, clinical or demographic variables in those patients who maintained sinus rhythm post cardioversion and those who experienced AF recurrence. This information was assessed in order to recommend an optimal follow-up strategy.

The results of studies were reported only where a particular electrophysiological, radiological, clinical or demographic variable had been stratified into meaningful value ranges and the measurement of recurrence made over a specific follow-up period.

Studies that had follow-up periods of less than 1 week or that considered only specialist investigations, such as signal-averaged ECG recording, were excluded. Echocardiographic risk factors for AF recurrence are reported elsewhere (see section 4.3).

12.2.2 Evidence statements

Twelve studies reporting the proportion of patients with recurrent AF at different intervals following successful cardioversion are as shown in Table 12.1.

	Study	N	Patients	Prior CV	Period	Recurrence (%)
Table 12.1 Percentage of patients with AF recurrence following cardioversion						
(2++)	Bollmann et al, 2003[327]	42	Recurrent	Yes	0.5	31
(2+)	Roijer et al, 2001[43]	62	Lone	No	1	32
(2+)	Dittrich et al, 1989[328]	65	Recurrent	No	1	31
(2+)	Duytschaever et al, 1998[46]	85	Recurrent	Yes	3.25	31
(2++)	Dmochowska-Perz et al, 2002[49]	112	Recurrent	Yes	6	55
(2++)	Aytemir et al, 1999[329]	74	Persistent	NR	6	42
(2+)	Okcun et al, 2002[330]	110	Recurrent	Yes	6	48
(2+)	Dittrich et al, 1989[328]	65	Recurrent	No	6	42
(2++)	Dogan et al, 2004[44]	64	Recurrent	No	6	44
(2++)	Guo et al, 2003[331]	60	Persistent	Yes	6	77
(2++)	Antonielli et al, 2002[42]	186	Recurrent	Yes	12	51
(2+)	Berry et al, 2001[332]	88	Recurrent	Yes	12	63
(2+)	Arnar and Danielsen, 1996[47]	44	Recurrent	Yes	12	43
(2+)	Paraskevaidis et al, 2005[50]	61	Lone	Yes	12	61
(2++)	Perez et al, 1997[333]	75	Recurrent	Yes	12	53

Prior CV = whether or not the patients enrolled in the study included those in whom a previous attempt at cardioversion had been performed.
Period = elapsed time since successful cardioversion (months).
Recurrence = percentage of patients with recurrent AF.

Up to 1 month following cardioversion, no significant differences have been found in any of the following pre-cardioversion factors in terms of the incidence of AF recurrence:
* presence of underlying heart disease[327] (2++) or cardiomegaly[208] (2+)
* gender[43] (2+)
* age greater than 70 years[43] (2+)
* AF duration of less than 2 weeks[43] (2+)
* use of antiarrhythmic drugs[43] (2+).

At approximately 3 months following cardioversion, no significant differences have been found in any of the following pre-cardioversion factors for the incidence of AF recurrence:[46] (2+)

- presence of underlying heart disease
- gender
- age greater than 70 years.

However, duration of AF of less than 12 months was found to be associated with an increased likelihood of maintaining sinus rhythm.[46] (2+)

At 6 months following cardioversion, the following pre-cardioversion factors have been found to be associated with an increased incidence of AF recurrence:

- a history of recurrent AF[49] (2++)
- chronic-obstructive pulmonary disease[330] (2+)
- heart failure.[49,330] (2++)

One study[44] found an AF duration of less than 5 days to be predictive of sinus rhythm maintenance at 6 months with sensitivity of 79% and specificity of 96% (2++). Another study[331] found AF duration to be significantly associated with incidence of AF recurrence when measured as a continuous variable, but not when dichotomised at 1 year. (2++)

Out of five studies[44,328–331] considering the association between gender and AF recurrence, only one[328] found a significantly higher proportion of men with AF recurrence at 6 months. (2++)

At 6 months following cardioversion, no significant differences have been found in any of the following pre-cardioversion factors in terms of the incidence of AF recurrence:

- age greater than 60 years[330] (2+)
- presence of any comorbid heart disease[44,331] (2+)
- presence of ischaemic heart disease[44,329–331] (2++), valvular heart disease[44] (2+) or cardiomegaly[334] (2+)
- presence of hypertension[44,329–331] (2++)
- presence of diabetes.[330] (2+)

At 12 months following cardioversion the following pre-cardioversion factors have been found to be associated with an increased incidence of AF recurrence:

- cardiomegaly[335] (2+)
- AF duration of more than 1 week.[42] (2+)

One study[335] reported a reduced risk of AF recurrence at 12 months among those patients in whom cardioversion was successful using only amiodarone prior to scheduled electrical cardioversion, compared with those in whom electrical cardioversion was required in addition to amiodarone (multivariate RR 0.075; 95% CI 0.01 to 0.54). (2++)

At 12 months following cardioversion the following pre-cardioversion factors have not been found to be associated with an increased incidence of AF recurrence:

- AF duration of more than 12 months[335] (2+) or 1 month[333] (2++)
- presence of ischaemic heart disease[42,333] or prior MI[42] (2++)
- presence of diabetes[42] (2++)
- presence of hypertension[42,333] (2++)
- gender.[50,333] (2++)

12.2.3 From evidence to recommendations

In terms of the incidence of recurrent AF, approximately one third of patients will relapse back to AF within the first month following successful cardioversion,[43,44,327,328] increasing to approximately half at 1 year.[42,47,50,332,333] There was not a large difference in the proportion of those reverting back to AF between 6 months and 1 year.

This suggests the need for routine follow-up for assessment at 1 month and 6 months following cardioversion. Those found still to be in sinus rhythm at 6 months could be discharged from secondary care and advised to attend primary care if symptoms re-occur.

A management strategy formulated prior to discharge from secondary care and shared with the patient's GP would be helpful in maintaining continuity of care.

The evidence was not considered strong enough to allow for the identification of specific patients in whom an alternative follow-up strategy would be beneficial.

It was agreed that the 1-month follow-up needs to be performed by a suitably trained healthcare professional.

In addition to assessing for relapse to AF, during each follow-up the clinician can take the opportunity to review:

* any comorbid factors (eg heart failure, hypertension)
* any adverse effects related to cardioversion (eg skin burns, thromboembolism)
* drug therapies (eg proarrhythmia from antiarrhythmic drugs, or bleeding from anticoagulation).

Furthermore, where a patient has relapsed to AF a decision needs to be made on whether an early attempt at a second cardioversion is appropriate or a rate-control strategy is more appropriate.

RECOMMENDATIONS

R60 Following successful cardioversion of AF routine follow-up to assess the maintenance of sinus rhythm should take place at 1 month and 6 months. D

R61 At the 1-month follow-up the frequency of subsequent reviews should be tailored to the individual patient taking into account comorbidities and concomitant drug therapies. D

R62 At each review the clinician should take the opportunity to re-assess the need for, and the risks and benefits of, continued anticoagulation. D(GPP)

R63 At 6 months, if patients remain in sinus rhythm and have no other need for hospital follow-up, they should be discharged from secondary care with an appropriate management plan agreed with their GP. D

R64 Patients should be advised to seek medical attention if symptoms recur. D(GPP)

R65 Any patient found at follow-up to have relapsed into AF should be fully re-evaluated for a rate-control or rhythm-control strategy (see section 6.3). D(GPP)

12.3 Referral

The purpose of this section is to identify which patients with AF might benefit from specialist investigations or interventions, but not to compare or contrast them with one another.

The most common reason for referral for specialist investigation or intervention is failed medical therapy due to antiarrhythmic drug intolerance or ineffectiveness. Secondly, those who may have an underlying electrophysiological problem, such as a pre-excitation syndrome due to an accessory pathway (eg Wolff–Parkinson–White syndrome) or those with focal AF, are commonly referred for pulmonary vein isolation. However, this procedure carries a small risk of pulmonary vein stenosis. Also, those with a family history of AF (familial AF)[336] may require specialist assessment. In addition, elderly patients may have sinus node disease that is associated with paroxysmal AF. Some[337] but not all[338] studies suggest a reduction in AF by atrial or physiological pacing. Pacemaker therapy in AF is also indicated for symptomatic low heart rates. Arrhythmia surgery, such as themaze operation, or less frequently, the corridor procedure, may be undertaken as a primary procedure – although uncommonly in the UK – or during associated cardiac surgery (eg mitral valve surgery).[339–341]

In drug-resistant, poorly tolerated AF, atrioventricular junction (AVJ) catheter ablation is an option.[342] A recent meta-analysis[343] of before-after studies in AVJ ablation and pacing showed a beneficial effect in terms of symptom severity, exercise tolerance, cardiac physiology and function, as well as hospital admissions. However, 'ablate and pace' carries a small risk of sudden death.[344,345]

Using technology similar to implantable cardioverter-defibrillators for ventricular arrhythmias, an atrial defibrillator (atrioverter) re-establishes sinus rhythm and reduces recurrences of persistent AF.[346] There is conflicting evidence on the tolerability of atrial defibrillators and of the risk of ventricular proarrhythmia.

12.3.1 Methodological introduction

Studies were included if either:

- a comparison was made between a medical treatment strategy that involved the use of either pharmacological intervention and/or electrical cardioversion (internal or external) and other device or procedure-based treatments, or
- the study compared the safety or efficacy of other device or procedure-based treatments or investigations between different patient subgroups (defined by either demographic, clinical or physiological characteristics).

Studies that compared two device- or procedure-based treatments (for example, two variants of the maze procedure) were not considered.

The following categories of device or procedure-based treatments were included:

- pulmonary vein isolation
- pacemaker therapy
- arrhythmia surgery
- AVJ catheter ablation
- atrial defibrillators.

The majority of studies not involving concomitant cardiac surgery included only medically-refractory patients. Such patients are defined in this report by: an explicit report of refractoriness in the study inclusion criteria; reported resistance to a mean of at least two antiarrhythmic drugs; or the report of patients experiencing intolerable symptoms associated with AF, either in terms of severity or (in the case of paroxysmal AF) frequency of episodes.

12.3.2 Evidence statements

▷ Pulmonary vein isolation

One study[347] comparing pulmonary vein isolation (PVI) with amiodarone therapy in a population of amiodarone-naïve patients with medically-refractory non-valvular recurrent AF found PVI to be associated with a higher prevalence of sinus rhythm at 12 months (p=0.03) and improved quality of life (p=0.048). (1+)

One study[348] in a population of relatively young (mean age 54 years) patients with recurrent AF (mostly PAF) with no previous use of antiarrhythmic drugs found that PVI was associated with higher rates of sinus rhythm maintenance at 12 months than pharmacological therapy with antiarrhythmic drugs (87% versus 37%; p<0.001) (1+). Those patients undergoing PVI also had fewer hospital admissions than those treated with drugs (9% versus 54%; p<0.001) (1+). In terms of quality of life, PVI was associated with a greater improvement in the following Short-Form 36 health survey subscales than drug therapy: (1+)

- general health
- physical functioning
- role physical
- bodily pain.

The study reported comparable efficacy between PVI and drug therapy in all other aspects of quality of life.

Two studies[349,350] found increasing age to be significantly associated with an increased incidence of AF recurrence following PVI (2+). However, another study[351] in a population with paroxysmal lone AF did not find age to be a significant independent predictor. (2+)

The results of one study[352] in patients with medically-refractory AF and a history of isthmus-mediated atrial flutter found men less likely to maintain sinus rhythm following PVI (2+). Another study[351] found no effect of gender and a successful outcome at 3 months. (2+)

Three studies[349,352,353] found that those with medically-refractory paroxysmal AF are more likely to maintain sinus rhythm following PVI than those with medically-refractory non-paroxysmal AF (2+). Those with medically-refractory paroxysmal AF were also found to be more likely to benefit from PVI than those with persistent AF in terms of overall treatment success (restoration and maintenance of sinus rhythm or significant improvement in symptoms at 5 months).[353] (2+)

One study[350] found that those with medically-refractory lone paroxysmal AF are more likely to benefit from PVI than those with comorbid paroxysmal AF in terms of prevalence of sinus rhythm at 1 month (2+). The results for other populations with medically-refractory lone AF is unclear.[349,352] (2+)

Those without a history of paroxysmal AF[353] or hypertension,[354] a left atrial diameter less than 40 mm[350] and normal left ventricular function[355] are more likely to benefit from PVI in terms of the maintenance of sinus rhythm. (2+)

▷ Pacemaker therapy

One crossover study[356] found that bi-atrial pacing was associated with a significant reduction in the amount of time spent in AF over 3 months compared with no pacing (1+). A similar result was found for right-atrial pacing alone (1+). However, no significant difference was found in terms of the frequency of AF episodes. (1+)

One small study[357] found no difference in the prevalence of structural heart disease among those maintaining sinus rhythm and those with AF recurrence following successful internal cardioversion and pacing of patients with permanent AF (63% versus 100%). (2+)

▷ Arrhythmia surgery

One study[358] of patients with AF undergoing a combined cardiac procedure with a modified maze procedure using cryoablation had a higher prevalence of sinus rhythm in the acute postoperative period compared with those undergoing cardiac procedures without any concomitant antiarrhythmic surgery (84% versus 6%; p<0.0001) (2+). The modified maze procedure was also associated with longer intubation and recovery times, as well as higher pulmonary artery and central venous blood pressure (2+). In the long term, the antiarrhythmia surgery was also associated with an improved NYHA grade. (2+)

Six studies[359–364] found that combining mitral valve procedures with antiarrhythmia surgery (the maze procedure or variants thereof), was more effective in restoring and maintaining sinus rhythm than mitral valve surgery alone for at least 3 years postoperatively. (1+)

One study[362] found the combination of mitral valve surgery and the maze procedure to be ineffective in improving any echocardiographically detected measure of cardiac physiology (including LVEF and left atrial diameter) compared with mitral valve surgery alone over 3 months and 12 months postoperatively (1+). Another study[363] found a similar result in NYHA grade over the same period. (1+)

One study[358] in a population with a mean duration of AF of approximately 8 years found the combination of mitral valve surgery and a modified maze procedure using cryoablation to be effective in reducing the cardiothoracic and the left atrial diameter compared with mitral valve surgery alone. (2+)

One study[362] found no differences in exercise tolerance between those patients undergoing combined mitral valve and maze surgery and those undergoing mitral valve surgery alone (1+). Another study[363] found a similar result, with the exception of maximum workload which was higher in those undergoing the maze procedure. (1+)

No significant beneficial effect of combining the maze procedure with cardiac surgery has been reported in terms of either quality of life[362] or mortality[364] at 12 months (1+). However, there is limited evidence[360] to suggest a reduction in adverse vascular events (stroke or anticoagulated-related bleeding events). (2+)

One study[365] found that combining mitral valve procedures with the corridor procedure resulted in more effective ventricular rate control than mitral valve surgery alone. (2+)

LAA filling velocity less than 20 cm/sec,[366] a duration of AF more than 10 years,[366] an enlarged left atrium[366–368] and an F wave less than 1 mm[368] are all associated with a reduced likelihood of sinus rhythm restoration and maintenance during the early postoperative period following combined cardiac surgery with PVI. (2+)

An enlarged left atrium has also been found to be associated with a longer time taken to revert to sinus rhythm following combined mitral valve surgery with the maze procedure,[369] as well as a longer time taken for the restoration of atrial contractile function in those in whom sinus rhythm was restored.[370] (2+)

It is unclear whether an enlarged left atrium is associated with a reduced likelihood of AF recurrence in the longer term after combined cardiac and antiarrhythmic surgery[369–371] (2+). However, one study[372] found a left atrial diameter of less than 57.8 mm and a left-atrial area of less than 56.25 cm^2 to have some degree of power in predicting the maintenance of sinus rhythm at 38 months following combined mitral valve surgery with the maze procedure. (2+)

One study[367] reported that the sensitivity and specificity of the regression equation 1.39-(0.387GLA)-(0.01AFD)-(0.007Age), where values over 0.843 predict postoperative sinus rhythm, was 73.2% and 88.9%, respectively (2+) (Note that GLA = 1 for the presence of a giant left atrium, 0 otherwise, and AFD is the duration of AF). However, the expression has not been validated prospectively in a separate cohort of patients.

▷ Atrioventricular junction ablation

Compared with continued pharmacological therapy, AVJ ablation is associated with a significant reduction in the number of hospital admissions[373,374] (1+), as well as the incidence of CHF.[374] (2+)

Three studies[342,373,374] found that AVJ ablation was more effective in reducing the overall severity of symptoms of AF compared with continued pharmacological treatment. (1+)

Four studies[342,373–375] are consistent in demonstrating a reduction in all symptoms commonly associated with AF, with the exception of syncope and resting dyspnoea, following AVJ ablation compared with continued pharmacological treatment (1+). However, two studies[342,375] failed to find any significant improvement in terms of overall quality of life. (1+)

The results of one study[374] in a population with lone AF found a difference in mean NYHA grade between AVJ ablation and pharmacological treatment in favour of AVJ ablation (2+). A consistent result was also found in a population with paroxysmal AF,[373] although the difference was not significant (1+). Another study[342] found no significant difference in terms of left-ventricular fractional shortening (LVFS). (1+)

One study[373] found that 24% of patients who underwent AVJ ablation developed permanent AF within 6 months, compared with no patients who continued pharmacological treatment (p=0.04) (1+). Another study[376] reported that those older than 75 years or those with comorbid cardiovascular disease are at an increased risk of developing permanent AF following AVJ ablation. (2+)

▷ Atrial defibrillator

The use of an atrial defibrillator with the defibrillator function activated is associated with a reduced burden of AF and a reduction in the number of hospital admissions compared with when the defibrillator function is de-activated[377] (2+). No significant association has been reported between the degree of patient acceptance of the implantation and use of an atrial defibrillator and patient age, gender, or the number of cardioversions performed pre-implantation.[378,28]

12.3.3 From evidence to recommendations

▷ Pulmonary vein isolation

From the evidence, it was noted that patients with the following characteristics may benefit from referral for PVI:
- patients who were resistant to pharmacological treatment
- younger rather than older patients or
- those with lone AF.

It was recognised that many of these patients may have focal AF secondary to a pulmonary vein foci and for those patients PVI may be a useful procedure.

▷ Pacemaker therapy

Other than recognised indications for pacemaker implantations such as sinus node disease, symptomatic bradycardia and chronotropic incompetence, no evidence was found to specifically identify other patients with AF who should be referred for pacemaker implantation.

▷ Arrhythmia surgery

Other than patients undergoing concomitant cardiac surgery (eg mitral valve surgery), there was no evidence to specifically identify patients for referral for arrhythmia surgery other than those who had failed other treatment options.

▷ AVJ catheter ablation

It was concluded that this technique was effective for patients with medically refractive paroxysmal AF, especially in the absence of any cardiac comorbidity.

▷ Atrial defibrillators

This technique was considered to be useful in patients with recurrent persistent AF but it should not be used in those with paroxysmal AF.

RECOMMENDATIONS

R66   Referral for further specialist intervention (for example, pulmonary vein isolation, pacemaker therapy, arrhythmia surgery, AVJ catheter ablation or use of atrial defibrillators) should be considered in the following patients:

- those in whom pharmacological therapy has failed   B
- those with lone AF   B
- those with ECG evidence of an underlying electrophysiological disorder (eg Wolff–Parkinson–White syndrome).   C

R67   The reasons for referral for specialist intervention should be explained and discussed with the patient.   D(GPP)

Appendix A:
Health economics modelling

The GDG selected a number of questions for which they felt more detailed health economic input would be useful. The following three areas were given priority:

- Economic analysis of the routine use of echocardiography versus selective use in clinical practice (routine ECHO model).
- Cost-effectiveness analysis of using TOE-guided CV in patients presenting with AF lasting for more than 48 hours for the presence of thrombi before cardioversion compared with conventional 3 to 4 weeks of anticoagulation (TOE model).
- The cost effectiveness of warfarin administration in AF patients, particularly the elderly (warfarin model).

No additional modelling was performed in the guideline on these topics for the reasons outlined below.

Routine ECHO model

When the model was presented to the GDG for discussion, the group were uncomfortable with the number of assumptions required for the model and the data sources used to obtain these. The GDG felt that the need to obtain health economics evidence for routine ECHO had been superseded, since routine ECHO is not going to be recommended. The recommendation for ECHO would be based on risk stratification and clinical criteria. The group voted to move on to the next topic for modelling.

TOE model

The health economist advised that a complex model was required to overcome limitations of the ACUTE trial. The technical team felt it would be difficult to populate this model with reliable data and were wary that the GDG would not be comfortable with a large number of assumptions. The project executive, aware of time constraints, advised that a rapid costing of the ACUTE trial was the only feasible option. Guidance was sought from health economist Jo Lord who advised that the costing of the ACUTE trial would be a misleading enterprise. The main concern was that the trial fails to establish the clinical superiority of the TOE strategy compared with the conventional anticoagulation strategy. A model designed on those data would have to incorporate an increase in mortality with TOE-guided CV. For this reason it was difficult to justify the rationale for conducting this cost-effectiveness analysis. Because of this, the TOE-guided CV model was not pursued.

Warfarin model

A review of the published cost-effectiveness literature was undertaken for this area prior to undertaking the modelling exercise. A large number of studies were identified (N=8) and thus it was agreed that there was sufficient literature to answer the question and no further analysis was required.

Appendix B:
Stroke risk stratification models

Stroke risk stratification models

Ref no.	Criteria (year)	Type	IV	EV	Low-risk criteria	Medium-risk criteria	High-risk criteria
[379]	ACCP 1 (1998)	1°/2°	No	Yes	No medium or high-risk factors	Diabetes coronary artery disease Thyrotoxicosis Age 65 to 75 years	Age >75 years History of hypertension Moderate–severe LV systolic dysfunction (by echocardiography)
[202]	ACCP 2 (2004)	1°/2°	No	No	No medium or high-risk factors	Age 65 to 75 years	Prior stroke/TIA or systemic embolism Age >75 years Moderate–severe LV systolic dysfunction (by echocardiography) Diabetes Hypertension
[168]	AFI 1 (1994)	1°/2°	Yes	Yes	No risk factors	Previous stroke or TIA History of hypertension History of diabetes Age >65 years	
[294]	AFI 2 (1999)+	1°/2°	No	No	Age <65 with no history of embolism, hypertension, diabetes, or other clinical risk factors	Age <65 with clinical risk factors: diabetes, hypertension, peripheral arterial disease, ischaemic heart disease. Age >65 not in high-risk group	Previous stroke or TIA Age ≥75 years AND hypertension and/or diabetes Clinical evidence of valve disease, heart failure, thyroid disease, and/or impaired left ventricular function on echocardiography
[28]	AFI 3 (2003)	1°/2°	Yes	Yes	No risk factors	Previous stroke or TIA Treated hypertension OR systolic blood pressure ≥160 mm Hg Previous MI OR angina Diabetes	
[295]	AHA/ ACC/ESC (2001)	1°/2°	No	No	No risk factors	Age ≥75 years Age >60 years with diabetes Age >60 years with coronary artery disease Heart failure (clinically determined) OR LVEF <35% Thyrotoxicosis Hypertension	
[296]	CHADS2 (2001)*	1°/2°	No	Yes	Score = 0	Score = 1 to 2	Score >2

continued

Stroke risk stratification models – *continued*

Ref no.	Criteria (year)	Type	IV	EV	Low-risk criteria	Medium-risk criteria	High-risk criteria
285	EAFT (1995)	2°	Yes	No	No risk factors	*Less than 3 risk factors:* • Previous (non-cerebrovascular) thromboembolism • Systolic blood pressure >160 mm Hg • Ischaemic heart disease • Cardiomegaly (CTR >50% by X-ray) • AF duration >1 year • At least one visible ischaemic cerebral lesion by CT scan	*3 or more risk factors:* • Previous (non-cerebrovascular) thromboembolism • Systolic blood pressure >160 mm Hg • Ischaemic heart disease • Cardiomegaly (CTR >50% by X-ray) • AF duration >1 year • At least one visible ischaemic cerebral lesion by CT scan
283	Framingham (2003)**	1°/2°	Yes	Yes	0–7	8–13	14–31
287	SPAF 1 (1992)	1°/2°	Yes	No	No risk factors	*Exactly 1 risk factor:* Previous thromboembolism History of hypertension Recent congestive heart failure	*More than 1 risk factor:* Previous thromboembolism History of hypertension Recent congestive heart failure
290	SPAF 2 (1995)	1°/2°	Yes	No	No risk factors	Previous thromboembolism Systolic blood pressure >160 mm Hg Recent episode of congestive heart failure OR LVFS ≤25% Female AND age >75 years	
282	SPAF 3 (1998)	1°	No	Yes	No risk factors	History of hypertension	Previous stroke or TIA or systemic embolism Systolic blood pressure >160 mm Hg Recent episode of congestive heart failure OR LVFS ≤25% Female AND age >75 years
192	SPAF 4 (1999)	1°/2°	Yes	No	No risk factors	Hypertension AND age ≤75 years Diabetes	Previous stroke or TIA Systolic blood pressure >160 mm Hg Hypertension AND age >75 years Female AND age >75 years
281	SPAF 5 (1999)	1°	Yes	No	No risk factors	Hypertension AND age ≤75 years Diabetes	Systolic blood pressure >160 mm Hg Hypertension AND age >75 years Female AND age >75 years

+AFI2 [294] was based on the initial AFI1 [168] risk stratification, but refined for a Birmingham primary care population by the AF Clinical Effectiveness Topic Group on behalf of the Birmingham Effectiveness Group, commissioned by Birmingham Health Authority. This was then implemented (31/8/97) as *Clinical Management in General Practice Guidelines* of the Birmingham Medical Audit Advisory Group and as a pan-Birmingham audit project in primary care by the Birmingham Health Authority.

*The CHADS2 system is based on the AFI1 and SPAF1 risk criteria, and assigns one point to CHF, hypertension, age >75, diabetes mellitus and two points to a previous stroke or TIA;

**Framingham 2003 assigned points to incremental increases in age (0 to 10 points) and blood pressure (0 to 3 points), and 6 points for being female, 5 points for diabetes and 6 points for a previous stroke or TIA. Risk stratification was made for CHADS2 and Framingham 2003 based on expected incidence of <2%, 2 to 6%, and >6% for low, medium and high-risk patients, respectively (using original cohort data).

Appendix C:
Clinical questions and search strategies

The table below lists all of the systematic reviews of the relevant literature that were performed as part of the development process of this guideline. In each case the section number of this guideline is given where the results of the systematic review are presented, along with the clinical question asked, and the corresponding search strategy used.

Section number	Question wording	Study type filters used	Databases and years
4.1	In patients with diagnosed AF (including those presenting with stroke), what are the frequencies of the presenting symptoms?	All study types including hospital- and population-based	Medline 1966–2005 Embase 1980–2005 Cochrane 1800–2005 Cinahl 1982–2005
4.2	In patients with suspected AF based on an irregular pulse, how accurate is an ECG in diagnosing AF?	Diagnosis	Medline 1966–2005 Embase 1980–2005 Cochrane 1800–2005 Cinahl 1982–2005
4.3	In which patients should echocardiography be performed to identify underlying structural/functional heart disease?	Diagnosis	Medline 1966–2005 Embase 1980–2005 Cochrane 1800–2005 Cinahl 1982–2005
4.4	In patients with suspected intermittent AF, how effective is ambulatory ECG rather than event ECG in diagnosing AF?	Diagnosis	Medline 1966–2005 Embase 1980–2005 Cochrane 1800–2005 Cinahl 1982–2005
5.1	Does electrical conversion versus pharmacological conversion affect rates of thromboembolism, quality of life, exercise capacity, failure rates?	All study types	Medline 1966–2005 Embase 1980–2005 Cochrane 1800–2005 Cinahl 1982–2005
5.2	In patients with persistent AF, is amiodarone better than a) flecainide or b) propafenone for use in cardioversion?	Systematic reviews, RCTs and comparative studies	Medline 1966–2005 Embase 1980–2005 Cochrane 1800–2005 Cinahl 1982–2005
5.2	In patients with AF is amiodarone better than sotalol for use in cardioversion?	Systematic reviews, RCTs and comparative studies	Medline 1966–2005 Embase 1980–2005 Cochrane 1800–2005 Cinahl 1982–2005
5.3	What is the safety and efficacy of the adjunctive administration of antiarrhythmic drugs for use in electrical cardioversion in comparison to electrical cardioversion without adjunctive antiarrhythmic drugs?	Systematic reviews, RCTs and comparative studies	Medline 1966–2005 Embase 1980–2005 Cochrane 1800–2005 Cinahl 1982–2005

continued

Clinical questions and search strategies – *continued*

Section number	Question wording	Study type filters used	Databases and years
5.4	Is a conventional anticoagulation strategy for elective cardioversion as effective as a transoesophageal echocardiogram plus anticoagulation?	Systematic reviews, RCTs, comparative studies and observational studies	Medline 1966–2005 Embase 1980–2005 Cochrane 1800–2005 Cinahl 1982–2005
6.1	In patients with AF, is flecainide or propafenone better than beta-blockers in maintaining sinus rhythm post cardioversion?	Systematic reviews, RCTs and comparative studies	Medline 1966–2005 Embase 1980–2005 Cochrane 1800–2005 Cinahl 1982–2005
6.1	In patients with AF, is amiodarone or sotalol better than beta-blockers in maintaining sinus rhythm post cardioversion?	Systematic reviews, RCTs and comparative studies	Medline 1966–2005 Embase 1980–2005 Cochrane 1800–2005 Cinahl 1982–2005
6.1	In patients with AF, is flecainide/propafenone better than amiodarone or sotalol in maintaining sinus rhythm post cardioversion?	Systematic reviews, RCTs and comparative studies	Medline 1966–2005 Embase 1980–2005 Cochrane 1800–2005 Cinahl 1982–2005
6.2	What is the efficacy of anticoagulation therapy versus placebo for stroke prevention in: a) paroxysmal AF b) permanent AF c) peri/post cardioversion to sinus rhythm d) acute/post-op AF e) peri/post stroke f) asymptomatic AF?	Systematic reviews, RCTs and comparative studies	Medline 1966–2005 Embase 1980–2005 Cochrane 1800–2005 Cinahl 1982–2005
6.2	What is the efficacy of anticoagulation therapy versus antiplatelet therapy for stroke prevention in: a) paroxysmal AF b) permanent AF c) peri/post cardioversion to sinus rhythm d) acute/post-op AF e) peri/post stroke?	Systematic reviews, RCTs and comparative studies	Medline 1966–2005 Embase 1980–2005 Cochrane 1800–2005 Cinahl 1982–2005
6.2	What is the efficacy of antiplatelet therapy versus placebo for stroke prevention in: a) paroxysmal AF b) permanent AF c) peri/post cardioversion to sinus rhythm d) acute/post-op AF e) peri/post stroke f) asymptomatic AF?	Systematic reviews, RCTs and comparative studies	Medline 1966–2005 Embase 1980–2005 Cochrane 1800–2005 Cinahl 1982–2005
6.3	In which patients with persistent AF does rate control result in improved mortality/morbidity/quality of life over rhythm control?	All study types	Medline 1966–2005 Embase 1980–2005 Cochrane 1800–2005 Cinahl 1982–2005
6.3	In which patients with persistent AF does rhythm control result in improved mortality/morbidity/quality of life over rate control?	All study types	Medline 1966–2005 Embase 1980–2005 Cochrane 1800–2005 Cinahl 1982–2005
7.1	In patients with permanent AF, what is the efficacy of rate-limiting calcium antagonists compared with digoxin in rate control?	Systematic reviews, RCTs and comparative studies	Medline 1966–2005 Embase 1980–2005 Cochrane 1800–2005 Cinahl 1982–2005

continued

Clinical questions and search strategies – *continued*

Section number	Question wording	Study type filters used	Databases and years
7.1	In patients with permanent AF, what is the efficacy of beta-blockers compared with digoxin in rate control?	Systematic reviews, RCTs and comparative studies	Medline 1966–2005 Embase 1980–2005 Cochrane 1800–2005 Cinahl 1982–2005
7.1	In patients with permanent AF, what is the efficacy of beta-blockers compared with rate-limiting calcium antagonists in rate control?	Systematic reviews, RCTs and comparative studies	Medline 1966–2005 Embase 1980–2005 Cochrane 1800–2005 Cinahl 1982–2005
7.1	In patients with permanent AF, what is the efficacy of rate-limiting calcium antagonists in combination with digoxin compared with rate-limiting calcium antagonists monotherapy in rate control?	Systematic reviews, RCTs and comparative studies	Medline 1966–2005 Embase 1980–2005 Cochrane 1800–2005 Cinahl 1982–2005
7.1	In patients with permanent AF, what is the efficacy of beta-blockers in combination with digoxin compared with beta-blocker monotherapy in rate control?	Systematic reviews, RCTs and comparative studies	Medline 1966–2005 Embase 1980–2005 Cochrane 1800–2005 Cinahl 1982–2005
7.2	What is the efficacy of anticoagulation therapy versus placebo for stroke prevention in: a) paroxysmal AF b) permanent AF c) peri/post cardioversion to sinus rhythm d) acute/post-op AF e) peri/post stroke f) asymptomatic AF?	Systematic reviews, RCTs and comparative studies	Medline 1966–2005 Embase 1980–2005 Cochrane 1800–2005 Cinahl 1982–2005
7.2	What is the efficacy of anticoagulation therapy versus antiplatelet therapy for stroke prevention in: a) paroxysmal AF b) permanent AF c) peri/post cardioversion to sinus rhythm d) acute/post-op AF e) peri/post stroke?	Systematic reviews, RCTs and comparative studies	Medline 1966–2005 Embase 1980–2005 Cochrane 1800–2005 Cinahl 1982–2005
7.2	What is the efficacy of antiplatelet therapy versus placebo for stroke prevention in: a) paroxysmal AF b) permanent AF c) peri/post cardioversion to sinus rhythm d) acute/post-op AF e) peri/post stroke f) asymptomatic AF?	Systematic reviews, RCTs and comparative studies	Medline 1966–2005 Embase 1980–2005 Cochrane 1800–2005 Cinahl 1982–2005
8.1	In patients with paroxysmal AF, is flecainide/propafenone better than beta-blockers in reducing the frequency of paroxysms?	Systematic reviews, RCTs and comparative studies	Medline 1966–2005 Embase 1980–2005 Cochrane 1800–2005 Cinahl 1982–2005
8.1	In patients with paroxysmal AF, is amiodarone or sotalol better than beta-blockers in reducing the frequency of paroxysms?	Systematic reviews, RCTs and comparative studies	Medline 1966–2005 Embase 1980–2005 Cochrane 1800–2005 Cinahl 1982–2005
8.1	In patients with paroxysmal AF, is flecainide/propefanone better than amiodarone or sotalol in reducing the frequency of paroxysms?	Systematic reviews, RCTs and comparative studies	Medline 1966–2005 Embase 1980–2005 Cochrane 1800–2005 Cinahl 1982–2005

continued

Clinical questions and search strategies – *continued*

Section number	Question wording	Study type filters used	Databases and years
8.2	In which patients should pill-in-the-pocket therapy be recommended?	All study types	Medline 1966–2005 Embase 1980–2005 Cochrane 1800–2005 Cinahl 1982–2005
9.1	In haemodynamically unstable patients presenting with acute AF, what is the best treatment strategy (ECV, PCV or acute (iv) rate control)?	Systematic reviews, RCTs, comparative studies, case control and observational studies	Medline 1966–2005 Embase 1980–2005 Cochrane 1800–2005 Cinahl 1982–2005
10.1, 10.2	What is the best treatment strategy (rate or rhythm control or no treatment) for patients with postoperative AF?	Systematic reviews, RCTs and comparative studies	Medline 1966–2005 Embase 1980–2005 Cochrane 1800–2005 Cinahl 1982–2005
10.1	Is the perioperative administration of antiarrhythmic drugs effective prophylaxis for post-operative AF?	Systematic reviews, RCTs and comparative studies	Medline 1966–2005 Embase 1980–2005 Cochrane 1800–2005 Cinahl 1982–2005
11.1	At the diagnosis of AF does immediate anticoagulation (comparison is absence of immediate Tx or later, delayed Tx) result in reduced rates of morbidity and mortality, without increasing pt anxiety, while still being cost effective?	Systematic reviews, RCTs, comparative studies, case control and cohort studies	Medline 1966–2005 Embase 1980–2005 Cochrane 1800–2005 Cinahl 1982–2005
11.5	In people with AF what are the risks of long-term oral anticoagulation administration as thromboprophylaxis?	Treatment outcomes, systematic reviews, RCTs, and comparative studies	Medline 1966–2005 Embase 1980–2005 Cochrane 1800–2005 Cinahl 1982–2005
11.6	In patients with AF, what are the risk factors associated with stroke/TIA and thromboembolism?	Risk, systematic reviews, RCTs, comparative studies and observational studies	Medline 1966–2005 Embase 1980–2005 Cochrane 1800–2005 Cinahl 1982–2005
12.1	In patients receiving anticoagulation therapy, is self-management using near-patient testing devices in primary care as effective as management using hospital lab testing?	Systematic reviews, RCTs, comparative studies, case control and observational studies	Medline 1966–2005 Embase 1980–2005 Cochrane 1800–2005 Cinahl 1982–2005 BNI 1985–2005
12.2	When should a cardioverted patient be followed up after cardioversion?	Systematic reviews, RCTs, comparative studies and observational studies	Medline 1966–2005 Embase 1980–2005 Cochrane 1800–2005 Cinahl 1982–2005
12.3	Which patients with AF benefit from referral to specialist services for non-pharmacological treatment or electrophysiological studies?	Systematic reviews, RCTs, comparative studies and observational studies	Medline 1966–2005 Embase 1980–2005 Cochrane 1800–2005 Cinahl 1982–2005

Note: The final cut-off date for all searches was 6th June 2005.

Appendix D:
Drug classification and licensing

Wherever appropriate, throughout this guideline recommendations have been formulated in terms of drug classes rather than individual drugs. The Vaughan-Williams system for classifying antiarrhythmic drugs such as flecainide (Class Ic) and amiodarone (Class III) has been used where appropriate.

In the case of rate-limiting calcium antagonists, certain drugs within this class may not be indicated for the treatment of AF. In particular, the rate-limiting calcium antagonist diltiazem hydrochloride is not indicated for AF, but nonetheless has a substantial evidence-base supporting its use.

Beta-blockers represent a wide range of agents, with different degrees of cardioselectivity. Certain beta-blockers may not be licensed specifically for AF. Sotalol is a beta-blocker that has additional Class III antiarrhythmic activity at high doses (240 to 480 mg/day). In UK practice, sotalol is often used at low doses (80 to 160 mg/day), which essentially acts in a similar manner to a standard beta-blocker (Class II) in terms of antiarrhythmic activity. In some patient groups (for example, those with a low body mass index or renal impairment), some Class III activity may even manifest at these low doses. In general, when used as a Class III antiarrhythmic agent, sotalol is often started at a dose of 80 mg twice daily for the first week and subsequently titrated to 160 mg twice daily or even higher doses after checking for adverse effects and QT prolongation on ECG.

Appendix E: Glossary of terms

Absolute risk reduction (ARR) The difference between the percentage incidence of adverse outcomes in the test group compared with the control group in a controlled trial, eg if the stroke rate in warfarin-treated patients is 2% compared with 5% in non-warfarin treated patients, warfarin is associated with an absolute risk reduction of 3%.

Accessory pathway An abnormal conduction circuit within the heart resulting in abnormal heart rhythms.

Adjusted dose The situation where the dosage of a drug is adjusted to attain a particular physiological value, eg the dosage of warfarin may be adjusted to attain a particular INR value.

Adverse event An event that occurs, normally as part of a pathological process or as an unintended consequence of a therapeutic intervention, which is considered to be of detrimental value to the patient in terms of their health or quality of life, eg the development of pulmonary fibrosis consequent to the long-term administration of amiodarone.

AF burden A measure of the degree to which the presence of AF has a detrimental effect on the patient's quality of life. It is normally measured either as the proportion of time spent in AF, or the number of AF episodes per unit time.

AF pathophysiology The pathological progression of AF in terms of the degeneration of the arrhythmia to a more sustained and/or symptomatic form, or the development of associated co-morbidities.

AF recurrence The recurrence of an episode of AF following one or more prior episodes of the arrhythmia in either its paroxysmal or persistent form.

AF subtype A subtype of AF based on its temporal pattern. AF subtypes are recent onset, paroxysmal, persistent and permanent.

Algorithm (in guidelines) A flowchart of the clinical decision pathway described in the guideline, where decision points and actions are represented by different shaped boxes and linked by arrows.

Ambulatory-ECG An ECG monitoring tool in which a continuous ECG recording is made while the patient remains able to walk around freely and pursue most normal daily activities.

Antiarrhythmic A drug or interventional procedure that has a therapeutic effect against cardiac arrhythmias.

Anticoagulation A form of thromboprophylaxis involving the use of anticoagulant drugs such as warfarin that inhibit the coagulation/clotting of blood.

Antiplatelet therapy A form of thromboprophylaxis involving the use of antiplatelet drugs (such as aspirin) that inhibit the formation of blood clots.

Antithrombotic therapy See 'thromboprophylaxis'.

Aortic plaque The deposits of atherosclerotic plaque within the aorta. The extent of aortic plaque is classified as 'simple', 'moderate' or 'complex'.

Aortic stenosis An abnormal narrowing of the aortic valve.

Arrhythmia An irregularity in the coordinated rhythm of the heart.

Arrhythmia surgery Antiarrhythmic surgical interventions to treat the abnormal heart rhythm, eg the 'maze' procedure, corridor operation. See also 'antiarrhythmic'.

Atrial arrhythmias Cardiac arrhythmias that originate in the atria. AF is an atrial arrhythmia. See also 'arrhythmia'.

Atrial contractile function A measurement of the contractile function of the atria. This is normally measured using echocardiography.

Atrial defibrillator See 'cardioverter defibrillator'.

Atrial fibrillation (AF) An atrial arrhythmia characterised by an absence of regular P waves on an electrocardiogram, and normally resulting in a fast ventricular response. See also 'atrial arrhythmia'.

Atrial filling fraction A measurement of the contractile function of the atria. This is normally measured using echocardiography.

Atrioventricular node ablation Use of energy (usually radiofrequency) to destroy tissue of the atrioventricular node to alter conduction of electrical signals through this part of the heart.

Atrioventricular-blocking drug A drug that inhibits the ability of the atrioventricular node to conduct electrical signals to the ventricles.

Audit See 'clinical audit'.

Binary A clinical variable or outcome is binary when it can only take on two possible values. In some cases variables that can take on more than two possible values, such as age, are dichotomised at a particular value to create a binary variables, such as 'under 65' and '65 or over'.

Bradycardia A slow heart beat. The occurrence of bradycardia is often recorded as an adverse event to some antiarrhythmic or chronotropic drugs. Such occurrences are referred to as bradycardic events.

Cardioembolic stroke An embolic stroke whose aetiology is presumed to be the embolisation of an intracardiac thrombus.

Cardiomegaly An abnormal enlargement of the heart. It is normally measured in terms of the cardiothoracic ratio from a chest X-ray or by measurement using echocardiography.

Cardiomemo An event recorder that records cardiac rhythm when activated by the patient.

Cardiothoracic ratio (CTR) See 'cardiomegaly'.

Cardioversion In the context of AF, cardioversion is the process of restoring normal sinus rhythm. There are two commonly used forms of cardioversion: electrical cardioversion and pharmacological cardioversion. The former involves the administration of a transthoracic electrical shock; the latter involves the administration of antiarrhythmic drugs.

Cardioverter defibrillator A defibrillator device that is implanted into the patient's chest to deliver an electrical shock to cardiovert episodes of AF. The device may be automated – automatic implanted cardioverter defibrillator – or patient-triggered. See also 'defibrillator'.

Case series Report of a number of cases of a given disease, usually covering the course of the disease and the response to treatment. There is no comparison (control) group of patients.

Case-control study Comparative observational study in which the investigator selects individuals who have experienced an event (for example, developed a disease) and others who have not (controls), and then collects data to determine previous exposure to a possible cause.

Cerebral infarction Damage to the brain following a reduction of blood supply to that area, resulting in a stroke.

Cerebrovascular disease Disease of the blood vessels within the brain. Cerebrovascular disease can be caused by blocked or otherwise damaged blood vessels and is the cause of strokes. See also 'stroke'.

Chronotropic In the context of pharmacology, the ability of a therapeutic intervention to control heart rate.

Chronotropic incompetence The inability of the body to appropriately alter heart rate during periods of physical exertion. See also 'chronotropic'.

Clinical audit A quality improvement process that seeks to improve patient care and outcomes through systematic review of care against explicit criteria and the implementation of change.

Clinically significant The result of a study is clinically significant if it is felt that the demonstrated difference in outcomes between the different arms of the study have the potential to inform and change clinical practice. A result may be statistically significant but not clinically significant, and vice versa.

Cohort study A retrospective or prospective follow-up study. Groups of individuals to be followed up are defined on the basis of presence or absence of exposure to a suspected risk factor or intervention. A cohort study can be comparative, in which case two or more groups are selected on the basis of differences in their exposure to the agent of interest.

Comparable In a statistical sense, a therapeutic intervention is said to be comparable to another if there is no statistically significant difference between them.

Compliance The extent to which a patient complies with a recommended treatment regimen.

Confidence interval (CI) A range of values which contains the true value for the population with a stated 'confidence' (conventionally 95%). The interval is calculated from sample data, and generally straddles the sample estimate. The 95% confidence value means that if the study, and the method used to calculate the interval, is repeated many times, then 95% of the calculated intervals will actually contain the true value for the whole population.

Confound The results of a study are confounded when there are thought to be other variables that were not controlled for in the study design, and where the effects of those variables on the results are unquantifiable and variable.

Congestive heart failure (CHF) Heart failure characterised by the inability of the heart to adequately support the body's physiological requirements.

Conventional anticoagulation The use of oral anticoagulation as a means of thrombo-prophylaxis, aiming for a target INR (usually 2.5, range 2–3) with monitoring and dose adjustment in an anticoagulation clinic. In the context of cardioversion, this is contrasted with the use of transoesophageal echocardiography to screen for the presence of thrombi and the use of parenteral anticoagulation prior to cardioversion, thus excluding the pre-cardioversion initiation of anticoagulation.

Coronary artery disease A disease which affects the arteries of the heart, normally through atherosclerosis of the coronary arteries, reducing the supply of blood to the heart and causing ischaemia and angina. See also 'ischaemic heart disease'.

Cost function A function that describes the relationship between the input prices such as labour costs, drugs, hospital stay and the quantity of outputs (health outcomes). It describes the opportunity cost, that is, what needs to be sacrificed in monetary terms in order to gain certain outcomes.

Cost effectiveness A measure of effectiveness that is relative to cost. For example, the cost effectiveness of antithrombotic therapy to prevent strokes may be measured in terms of the cost per stroke prevented. See also cost-effectiveness analysis and cost-effectiveness model.

Cost-effectiveness analysis An economic study design in which consequences of different interventions are measured using a single outcome, usually in natural units (for example, life-years gained, deaths avoided, heart attacks avoided, cases detected). Alternative interventions are then compared in terms of cost per unit of effectiveness.

Cost-effectiveness model An explicit mathematical framework, which is used to represent clinical decision problems and incorporate evidence from a variety of sources in order to estimate the costs and health outcomes.

Cost–utility analysis A form of cost-effectiveness analysis in which the units of effectiveness are quality-adjusted life-years (QALYS).

Coumarin derivative An anticoagulant drug that is derived from coumarin. Examples of coumarin derivatives include the anticoagulant warfarin.

Crossover study A study design in which the participants are first administered the control intervention, followed by the test intervention, or vice versa. In between these two study phases there is normally a wash-out period in the case of drug trials, so that the levels of the control or test drug falls to negligible amounts before the next phase of the study begins.

Cryoablation Use of cold energy ('freezing') to destroy tissue within the heart in order to alter conduction of electrical signals through this part of the heart.

CT scan Computed tomography scan, an imaging technique using X-rays.

Day case In the context of cardioversion, a day case refers to the discharge of patients following elective cardioversion on the same day on which they were admitted.

Decision analytic model/techniques A way of reaching decisions, based on evidence from research. This evidence is translated into probabilities and then into diagrams or decision trees that direct the clinician through a succession of possible scenarios, actions and outcomes.

Decision model A systematic framework of representing a clinical problem under conditions of uncertainty. It is used to determine the costs and health outcomes of a hypothetical patient cohort with disease of interest when they are treated with different clinical strategies.

Defibrillator In the context of AF, a device used to deliver the electrical shock used in electrical cardioversion.

Diagnostic accuracy The degree to which a diagnostic (or screening) tool or procedure is able to distinguish between cases and non-cases. See also 'sensitivity', 'specificity', 'negative predictive value' and 'positive predictive value'.

Diastolic Relating to the phase of the cardiac cycle where the chambers of the heart fill with blood prior to being pumped out during the subsequent systolic phase. See also 'systolic'.

Discounted survival See 'discounting'.

Discounting The process of converting the cost or benefits to be incurred or received at different points in the future to a present value so that they can be compared in commensurate units as if they all occur at the same point in time.

Dominance An intervention is said to dominate an alternative intervention if it is both more effective clinically and less costly.

Drug-eluting stents Special metallic devices which are placed within the coronary artery to reduce the likelihood of coronary stenosis recurring following angioplasty (balloon dilatation of the coronary artery). Drug eluting stents have special drugs within their structure that greatly reduce the recurrence of stenoses.

Dyspnoea Breathlessness.

Echocardiogram An examination of the heart using ultrasound-imaging techniques. An echocardiogram may be performed by placing the ultrasound device across the chest (transthoracic echocardiography), or by inserting it down the gullet to view the heart from behind (transoesophageal echocardiography).

Electrical cardioversion (ECV) See 'cardioversion'.

Electrocardiograph (ECG) A device which traces the electrical activity of the heart by recording the electrical potentials at electrodes placed at various locations around the chest. The recording produced by the electrocardiograph is referred to as an electrocardiogram.

Electrolyte abnormalities Abnormalities or an imbalance in one or more of the body's salts or other chemicals in the blood circulation.

Embolic The passage within the blood stream of a body (eg blood clot), which has formed somewhere and ends up elsewhere within the body (eg brain).

Endpoint In the context of study design, an endpoint is a pre-defined event or events whose occurrence represents the end of follow-up. A composite endpoint is one where more than one event is pre-defined, and the occurrence of any one of them represents the end of follow-up. A primary endpoint is the occurrence of the event, which is the main outcome of interest.

Event-ECG recorder An ECG recording device, which only produces an ECG recording when susceptible electrical activity is detected. It may be triggered automatically or by the patient upon the occurrence of symptoms. See 'cardiomemo'.

Exercise tolerance A measure of a patient's capacity for physical exertion.

Extra cellular fluid volume A term that refers to the fluid bathing the body's cells.

Focal AF AF secondary to a focus of abnormal cells (eg near the pulmonary veins) that can initiate AF.

Functional heart disease Abnormalities of cardiac function – either in systole or diastole.

Good practice point (GPP) Recommended good practice based on the clinical experience of the guideline development group in the absence of robust, published clinical evidence.

Grade (class) of recommendation All recommendations are assigned a grade (A, B, C, D or D(GPP)) according to the level of evidence the recommendation is based on (see 'level of evidence').

Guideline development group (GDG) The guideline development group agrees the clinical questions for the guideline, considers the evidence and develops the recommendations. The GDG membership is multidisciplinary comprising clinicians, patients and/or carers and technical experts.

Haemodynamic function An assessment of cardiac function.

Haemodynamic instability Where cardiac function is compromised so that the patient becomes clinically unstable.

Haemorrhagic death Death caused by a haemorrhagic event such as an intracranial haemorrhage.

Haemorrhagic stroke Stroke secondary to cerebral haemorrhage.

Haemorrhagic transformation The situation where there is bleeding into a (usually large) cerebral infarction, especially in the early phase of a stroke.

Health technology assessment (HTA) These consider the effectiveness, appropriateness and cost of technologies and are funded by the NHS Research and Development Division.

Heart failure See 'congestive heart failure'.

Heart murmur An audible sound with or without a stethoscope, which relates to abnormal flow within the heart or an abnormal communication within the circulatory system.

Heart rate The rate at which the heart performs a complete cycle of coordinated muscular contraction. It is measured in beats per minute (bpm).

Holter monitor An ambulatory ECG recording device.

Hyperadrenergic state Situations where there is abnormal circulating adrenaline (and similar hormones) and/or activation of the sympathetic nervous system eg 'fight or flight' reaction.

Hypertension Abnormally high blood pressure.

Hypotension Abnormally low blood pressure.

Incidence The rate at which an event occurs. Incidence normally measures the rate at which people within a population develop a particular disease or experience other adverse events.

Inconclusive A series of study results are inconclusive when the evidence of different studies do not conflict with each other, but nonetheless lack the strength to be able to reach a definite conclusion.

Incremental cost per QALY The additional cost incurred for each additional QALY. See also 'incremental cost-effectiveness ratio'.

Incremental cost-effectiveness ratio (ICER) A ratio obtained by dividing the incremental costs (cost difference) by the incremental benefits (outcome differences) for two interventions. This depicts the extra cost per unit of outcome. A decision will be made as to whether the additional cost per unit of outcome is worth paying for based on the decision-maker's willingness to pay.

Independent predictor A variable whose value predicts the occurrence of an event independent of the values of other variables.

Infarction An ischaemic lesion. Cerebral infarctions can result in stroke, and myocardial infarctions can result in a heart attack. See also 'myocardial infarction'.

Informed dissent The situation whereby a patient elects to abstain from receiving the optimal therapeutic intervention in the knowledge that this could cause them harm.

Inotropic Drugs that can stimulate the contraction of the heart.

Intention-to-treat analysis (ITT analysis) An analysis of the results of a clinical study in which the data are analysed for all study participants as if they had remained in the group to which they were randomised, regardless of whether or not they remained in the study until the end, crossed over to another treatment or received an alternative intervention.

Intermittent atrial fibrillation AF that is not sustained, but interrupted by periods of sinus rhythm. Intermittent AF is normally considered to apply to more patients than paroxysmal AF, since the periods of sinus rhythm in the former may be very brief and otherwise insignificant.

International normalised ratio (INR) A measure of the clotting ability of blood, usually following use of anticoagulant drugs. It is calculated as the ratio of the length of time it takes blood to clot over the time it would take the blood of a normal subject to clot.

Intracardiac Occurring within the chambers of the heart.

Intracranial haemorrhage A bleeding event within the brain, which may result in a haemorrhagic stroke.

Intubation Being intubated with a transoesophageal breathing tube connected to a mechanical ventilator.

Ischaemic heart disease Heart disease characterised by a reduced supply of blood to the heart. See also 'coronary artery disease'.

Ischaemic stroke Stroke caused by cerebral infarction.

Lacunar infarction Stroke secondary to blockage of the small vessels especially at the border of zones supplied by different arteries.

Left atrial appendage velocity A measurement of the blood flow within the left atrial appendage, usually on TEE.

Left bundle branch block (LBBB) A conduction abnormality of the heart due to impaired conduction down the left bundle of His.

Left ventricular dysfunction (LVD) Impaired function of the left ventricle.

Left ventricular ejection fraction (LVEF) The percentage of blood within the left ventricle that is ejected at each contraction.

Left ventricular end diastolic diameter (LVEDD) A measurement of the size of the heart on echo, referring to the internal dimension of the heart in diastole.

Left ventricular end systolic diameter (LVESD) A measurement of the size of the heart on echo, referring to the internal dimension of the heart in systole.

Left ventricular hypertrophy (LVH) Thickening of the heart muscle, usually secondary to hypertension, aortic valve narrowing etc.

Left ventricular shortening fraction (LVFS) A measure of left ventricular function on echo.

Level of evidence A code (eg 1++, 1+, 2++) linked to an individual study, indicating where it fits into the NICE hierarchy of evidence and how well it has adhered to recognised research principles.

Lone AF AF that occurs in the absence of any comorbid cardiovascular disease or other precipitants of AF.

Magnetic resonance imaging (MRI) A non-invasive imaging technique allowing detailed examination of the heart.

Management strategy The overarching plan on how to treat a particular patient. In the context of AF, there are two main management strategies – rate control and rhythm control.

Maximum workload A measure of exercise tolerance. See 'exercise tolerance'.

Medically refractory In the context of AF, a patient is medically refractory if successive trials of different drugs and attempts at cardioversion fail to adequately control the symptoms or pathophysiology of AF.

Meta-analysis A statistical technique for combining (pooling) the results of a number of studies that address the same question and report on the same outcomes to produce a summary result. The aim is to derive more precise and clear information from a large data pool. It is generally more reliably likely to confirm or refute a hypothesis than the individual trials.

Methodological limitations Features of the design or reporting of a clinical study which are known to be associated with risk of bias or lack of validity. Where a study is reported in this guideline as having significant methodological limitations, a recommendation has not been directly derived from it.

Mitral annular abnormalities Echo abnormalities of the mitral valve ring/annulus, such as mitral annular calcification.

Mitral regurgitation A backwards flow of blood through the mitral valve normally caused by a dysfunctional mitral valve disease. Mitral regurgitation is classified as 'mild', 'moderate' or 'severe'.

Mitral stenosis An abnormal narrowing of the mitral valve. It can be measured echocardiographically by the mitral valve area.

Mitral valve calcification Deposition of calcium on the mitral valve.

Mitral valve disease Common generic term for disease of the mitral valve.

Mitral valve prolapse Condition where one or more mitral valve leaflets do not appose correctly and there is backward movement of the valve into the atrium, leading to mitral regurgitation.

Mitral valvuloplasty Stretching of the mitral valve, at surgery or using a balloon technique.

Monotherapy In the context of drug therapy, the administration of a single drug for a particular indication.

Multivariate Involving multiple variables. See also 'univariate'.

Myocardial infarction (MI) Heart attack.

National Collaborating Centre for Chronic Conditions (NCC-CC) A partnership of the Clinical Effectiveness Forum for Allied Health Professions, the NHS Confederation, the Patient Involvement Unit at NICE, the Royal College of General Practitioners, the Royal College of Nursing, the Royal College of Physicians of London, the Royal College of Physicians' Patient and Carers Liaison Committee, the Royal College of Surgeons of England, and the Royal Pharmaceutical Society of Great Britain. Set up in 2000 to undertake commissions from NICE to develop clinical guidelines for the NHS.

National Institute for Health and Clinical Excellence (NICE) NICE is the independent organisation responsible for providing national guidance on the promotion of good health and the prevention and treatment of ill health.

National Service Framework (NSF) A series of reports recommending service levels and targets for particular disease groups in the UK.

Negative predictive value The proportion of individuals with a negative test result who do not have the disease.

Negative predictor A variable whose values are inversely related to the likelihood of an event occurring.

New York Heart Association (NYHA) Score A score graded between 1 and 4 that measures cardiac function. Those patients with a score of 4 are considered to have severe heart failure; those with a score of 1 are considered to have asymptomatic or mild heart failure.

Non-significant See 'statistical significance'.

Number needed to treat (NNT) The number of patients who must be treated to prevent a single occurrence of the outcome of interest, based on an average calculated from the available data.

Nurse-led cardioversion Practice where the cardioversion procedure is organised, performed and patient follow-up undertaken by specialist nurses.

Odds ratio (OR) A measure of treatment effectiveness. The odds of an event happening in the treatment group, expressed as a proportion of the odds of it happening in the control group. The 'odds' is the ratio of non-events to events.

Open-label In the context of study design, a study in which the physicians or investigators are not blinded to which patients are allocated to which treatment arm.

Pacing The situation where a device (a pacemaker) complements or replaces the natural conducting system of the heart.

Palpitations The experience of one's own heartbeat as an awareness of the heart beating or a thumping sensation originating in the chest.

Patent foramen ovale A 'hole in the heart' where there is a congenital connection between the left and right atria.

Percutaneous coronary intervention (PCI) Any procedure on the heart undertaken by insertion of a device (eg stent) through a small hole in an artery (eg radial artery, femoral artery).

Peripheral artery disease Atherosclerotic vascular disease involving the peripheral arteries.

Pharmacological cardioversion (PCV) See 'cardioversion'.

Pill-in-the-pocket A management strategy for paroxysmal AF involving the patient self-administering antiarrhythmic drugs only upon the onset of an episode of AF.

Platelet-thrombus Blood clot that is rich in platelets rather than fibrin.

Pneumonectomy Removal of whole or part of a lung.

Polypharmacy The administration of multiple drugs for one or more indications.

Pooled analysis The aggregation of patient data from multiple separate studies with the objective of increasing the likelihood of being able to detect significant associations that would otherwise have been missed.

Positive predictive value (PPV) The proportion of individuals with a positive test result who actually have the disease.

Precipitant A disease process, toxin, or physiological abnormality which is known to predispose towards development of AF. In many cases, AF precipitants may not be identifiable, in other cases there are identifiable precipitants such as heart failure or alcohol excess.

Pre-excitation syndrome A condition that can predispose to arrhythmia, due to an accessory pathway leading to early/premature excitation of part of the heart. Examples include Wolff–Parkinson–White syndrome and Lown–Ganong–Levine syndrome.

Prevalence The proportion of people within a population who have a particular disease.

Pro-arrhythmic Pre-disposing to the development of cardiac arrhythmias.

Prophylactic Having a preventative action against one or more adverse events.

Pulmonary vein isolation Procedure where ablation is used to create a scar that isolates the tissue of the pulmonary vein from the rest of the heart – thus, if a focus precipitating AF is from within the pulmonary veins, the abnormal electrical impulses cannot reach the heart.

Pulse palpation The act of feeling for, and counting, the pulse.

QT prolongation The prolongation of the QT interval on an electrocardiogram.

Quality of life A measure of a person's overall wellbeing, taking into consideration not only the physical morbidity associated with disease, but also how this detrimentally effects social and psychological functioning.

Quality-adjusted life-year (QALY) An index of survival that is adjusted to account for the patient's quality of life during this time. QALYs have the advantage of incorporating changes in both quantity (longevity/mortality) and quality (morbidity, psychological, functional, social and other factors) of life. Used to measure benefits in cost–utility analysis.

Randomised controlled trial (RCT) A comparative study in which participants are randomly allocated to intervention and control groups and followed up to examine differences in outcomes between the groups.

Rapid atrial fibrillation AF that is associated with a very fast heart beat.

Rate control The attempt to treat AF not through the restoration of sinus rhythm, but through the control of the ventricular rate and the management of stroke risk. See also 'rhythm control'.

Regression equation An equation that assigns weights (co-efficients) to different variables according to the degree to which they are able to predict the occurrence of a particular event or value.

Relative risk (RR) The number of times more likely or less likely an event is to happen in one group compared with another (calculated as the risk of the event in group A, divided by the risk of the event in group B).

Relative risk reduction (RRR) The percentage reduction in the relative risk gained by a particular therapeutic intervention in comparison to another. See also 'relative risk'.

Rhythm control The attempt to treat AF through the restoration and maintenance of sinus rhythm and the management of stroke risk. See also 'rate control'.

Right bundle branch block (RBBB) A conduction abnormality of the heart due to impaired conduction down the right bundle of His.

Risk stratification The process of allocating patients to different levels of risk of an adverse event occurring, based on their clinical or other characteristics.

Self-management In the context of anticoagulation, the process of the patient testing their own blood and making dose-adjustments where necessary.

Self-testing In the context of anticoagulation, the process of the patient testing their own blood and their treating physician recommending dose-adjustments where necessary.

Sensitivity The proportion of individuals classified as positive by the gold or reference standard, who are correctly identified by the study test.

Sensitivity analysis A technique used in economic evaluation or decision analysis to determine how and/or whether plausible changes in uncertain clinical or costing variables affect the main results of the analysis.

Side effect An adverse event that occurs because of a therapeutic intervention.

Significant association See 'statistical significance'.

Significant difference See 'statistical significance'.

Sinus rhythm The normal pattern of electrical activity (and subsequent muscular contraction) of the heart.

Specificity The proportion of individuals classified as negative by the gold (or reference) standard, who are correctly identified by the study test.

Spontaneous cardioversion The process of cardioversion that occurs in the absence of any therapeutic interventions.

Spontaneous echo contrast Smoke-like appearance within the chambers of the heart – usually on TOE – which indicates stasis of blood within the chamber.

Statistical significance A statistical association or difference between two or more variables that has less than a 5% chance of happening through the random concatenation of events is considered to be statistically significant.

Structural heart disease The presence of abnormalities of the heart valves, muscle, chambers etc.

Sudden cardiac death syndrome The condition whereby a patient dies suddenly and unexpectedly with no obvious precipitants.

Supervised management In the context of anticoagulation management, supervised management refers to the situation where a clinician determines any dose adjustments and takes blood measurements.

Supraventricular Pertaining to the atria, eg supraventricular arrhythmia is an abnormal heart rhythm originating in the atria.

Systematic review Research that summarises the evidence on a clearly formulated question according to a pre-defined protocol using systematic and explicit methods to identify, select and appraise relevant studies, and to extract, collate and report their findings. It may or may not use statistical meta-analysis.

Systemic emboli Emboli that has reached the systemic circulation, potentially causing a systemic embolism. See 'embolic'.

Systolic Relating to the phase of contraction of the chambers of the heart during which they eject blood following the diastolic phase. See also 'diastolic'.

Tachycardia-induced cardiomyopathy A form of cardiomyopathy (damage to the heart muscle cells) caused by an excessive heart rate.

Temporal pattern The pattern distinguishing between different subtypes of AF.

Thromboembolic stroke Thrombus that has travelled to the brain circulating leading to blockage of an artery and causing a stroke. See 'embolic', 'stroke'.

Thromboembolism The embolisation (disloading and transportation in the blood) of a thrombus.

Thromboprophylaxis The administration of antithrombotic therapy (anticoagulation, antiplatelet therapy) for the prevention of thrombus formation.

Thrombus Blood clot.

Thyrotoxicosis A disease caused by the hyperactivity of the thyroid glands.

TOE-guided cardioversion In the context of cardioversion, the management of peri-cardioversion thromboembolic risk through the use of transoesophageal echocardiography (TOE) to screen for intracardiac thrombi alongside parenteral anticoagulation. See also 'conventional anticoagulation'.

Torsades de pointes A type of ventricular arrhythmia, which is a polymorphic ventricular tachycardia characterised by 'twisting of points' and commonly associated with a prolonged QT interval on the ECG.

Transoesphageal echocardiography See 'echocardiogram'.

Transient ischaemic attack An ischaemic cerebral event which does not result in any disability or cognitive impairment beyond 24 hours.

Transthoracic echocardiography See 'echocardiogram'.

Treatment failure Failure of the prescribed drug regimen to work. Demonstrated by a lack of clinical improvement or reduction in arrhythmia, etc.

Univariate Pertaining to a single variable. See also 'multivariate'.

Valvular heart disease Diseases of heart valves, eg mitral valve disease.

Vascular death Death caused by a cardiovascular disease or adverse cardiovascular event such as an acute myocardial infarction.

Vascular disease Disease of the vascular system, including both coronary and peripheral blood vessels.

Vaughan-Williams A classification system of antiarrhythmic drugs, depending on whether the drugs activity is as a sodium-channel blocker (Class I), a beta-blocker (Class II), a repolarisation-prolonging agent (Class III), or a calcium-channel blocker (Class IV).

Ventricular arrhythmias Cardiac arrhythmias that originate in the ventricles. See also 'arrhythmia'.

Ventricular rate control See 'rate control'.

Volume loss A term that usually refers to the amount of blood lost.

Wall motion index (WMI) An echocardiographic measure of the contractile function of the ventricles.

Wash-out period A period between the different experimental phases of a crossover study to ensure that no significant traces of previously administered drugs are left in the body to confound the results.

Wolff–Parkinson–White syndrome (WPW) See 'pre-excitation syndrome'.

Appendix F: Stakeholders

The following are registered stakeholders in the development or validation of this guideline:

Black Country Cancer and Cardiac Network

Association of British Healthcare Industries

Association of the British Pharmaceuticals Industry

AstraZeneca UK Ltd

Bard Ltd

Bayer Healthcare Plc

Biotronik UK Ltd

Boehringer Ingelheim Ltd

Boston Scientific Limited

Bristol-Myers Squibb Pharmaceuticals Ltd

Caledonian Medical Ltd

CardioLogic Limited

Guidant Corporation

Johnson & Johnson Medical

Medtronic Limited

P.M.S (Instruments) Ltd

Roche Diagnostics Limited

Sanofi-Aventis

Sorin Group CRM

St Jude Medical UK Ltd

Takeda UK Limited

Bedfordshire and Hertfordshire NHS Strategic Health Authority

North East London Strategic Health Authority

Addenbrookes NHS Trust

Aintree Hospitals NHS Trust

Airedale General Hospital – Acute Trust

Barnsley Primary Care Trust

Blaenau Gwent Local Health Board

Bradford South & West Primary Care Trust

Burntwood, Lichfield and Tamworth Primary Care Trust

Cardiff and Vale NHS Trust

Chorley and South Ribble Primary Care Trust

City and Hackney Teaching Primary Care Trust

Conwy and Denbighshire NHS Trust

Conwy Local Health Board

Countess of Chester Hospital NHS Foundation Trust

Craven Harrogate and Rural District Primary Care Trust

Denbighshire Local Health Board

East and North Herts. NHS Trust

Greater Peterborough Primary Care Partnership-North Primary Care Trust

Guys & St Thomas' NHS Trust

Heart of England NHS Foundation Trust

Leeds North East Primary Care Trust

Leeds Teaching Hospitals NHS Trust

Liverpool PCTs Medicines Management Team

Luton and Dunstable Hospital NHS Trust

Maidstone and Tunbridge Wells NHS Trust

Mansfield District Primary Care Trust

Newcastle Primary Care Trust

Newcastle under Lyme Primary Care Trust

Newcastle upon Tyne Hospitals NHS Trust

North Bradford Primary Care Trust

North Cumbria Acute Hospitals NHS Trust

North East Lincolnshire Primary Care Trust

North Lincolnshire Primay Care Trust

North Tees Primary Care Trust

Northwest London Hospitals NHS Trust

Papworth Hospital NHS Trust

Princess Alexandra Hospital NHS Trust

Queen Elizabeth Hospital NHS Trust (Woolwich)

Queen Elizabeth NHS Trust (Norfolk)

Queen Victoria Hospital NHS Foundation Trust

Rotherham Primary Care Trust

Royal Brompton and Harefield NHS Trust

Royal United Hospital Bath NHS Trust

Salford Primary Care Trust

Sedgefield Primary Care Trust

Sheffield South West Primary Care Trust

Sheffield Teaching Hospitals NHS Trust

Sheffield West Primary Care Trust

South East Sheffield Primary Care Trust

Staffordshire Moorlans Primary Care Trust

Stockport Primary Care Trust

Tameside and Glossop Acute Services NHS Trust

The North West London Hospitals NHS Trust

Trafford Primary Care Trusts

University Hospital Birmingham NHS Trust

University Hospitals Coventry and Warwickshire NHS Trust

Vale of Aylesbury Primary Care Trust

Waveney Primary Care Trust

Wrightington Wigan and Leigh NHS Trust

Anticoagulation Europe

Arrhythmia Alliance

British Heart Foundation

Sudden Adult Death Trust

The Progressive Supranuclear Palsy (PSP Europe) Association

The Stroke Association

Association of British Neurologists

British Association for Nursing in Cardiac Care

British Cardiovascular Society

British Geriatrics Society

British Pacing and Electrophysiology Group

British Psychological Society

British Society for Haematology

British Society for Heart Failure

Central Liverpool Primary Care Trust

Cochrane Heart Group

Heartsave

Independent Healthcare Forum

NHS Direct

Primary Care Cardiovascular Society

Royal College of Anaesthetists

Royal College of General Practitioners

Royal College of General Practitioners
Wales

Royal College of Nursing

Royal College of Pathologists

Royal College of Physicians of Edinburgh

Royal College of Physicians of London

Royal Pharmaceutical Society of Great
Britain

Society and College of Radiographers

Society of Cardiothoracic Surgeons

The David Lewis Centre

The Royal Society of Medicine

UK Specialised Services Public Health
Network

Academic Cardiology

Cardiology Research Department of St
Barts Hospital

Society for Academic Primary Care

University of Birmingham, Department of
Primary Care and General Practice

British National Formulary

Commission for Social Care Inspection

Connecting for Health

Department of Health

Healthcare Commission

Medicines and Healthcare Products
Regulatory Agency (MHRA)

National Patient Safety Agency

National Public Health Service – Wales

NHS Health and Social Care Information
Centre

NHS Quality Improvement Scotland

PERIGON (formerly The NHS
Modernisation Agency)

Regional Public Health Group – London

Scottish Intercollegiate Guidelines Network

Welsh Assembly Government

Appendix G: Scope

Guideline title

Atrial fibrillation: the management of atrial fibrillation

▷ Short title

Atrial fibrillation

Background

The National Institute for Health and Clinical Excellence (NICE or 'the Institute') has commissioned the National Collaborating Centre for Chronic Conditions to develop a clinical guideline on AF for use in the NHS in England and Wales. This follows referral of the topic by the Department of Health and Welsh Assembly Government (see below). The guideline will provide recommendations for good practice that are based on the best available evidence of clinical and cost effectiveness.

The Institute's clinical guidelines will support the implementation of National Service Frameworks (NSFs) in those aspects of care where a framework has been published. The statements in each NSF reflect the evidence that was used at the time the framework was prepared. The clinical guidelines and technology appraisals published by the Institute after an NSF has been issued will have the effect of updating the framework.

Clinical need for the guideline

Atrial fibrillation (AF) is the most common sustained cardiac arrhythmia. The prevalence of AF increases with age and is the most common arrhythmia causing hospitalisation. In a UK cohort, the prevalence of AF was 8 per 1,000 in males, and 5 per 1,000 in females, with an incidence of 0.9 new cases per 1,000 patient years in males, and 0.2 new cases per 1,000 patient years in females. An increased incidence is associated with age, gender and the presence of other common diseases, including hypertension, heart failure, ischaemic heart disease, diabetes and peripheral artery disease.

AF is associated with a substantial mortality, and with morbidity and hospitalisation from stroke, heart failure, thromboembolism and impaired cognitive function. From a large follow-up study over 40 years, AF was associated with a 1.5 fold (male) to 1.9 fold (female) increased risk of mortality after adjustment for pre-existing cardiovascular disease.

As a common arrhythmia and a cause of substantial morbidity and mortality, AF has considerable implications for healthcare expenditure. Recently, the total cost of AF to the NHS in 2000 (using conservative 1995 prevalence figures) has been calculated to be £459 million or 0.97% of total expenditure. The cost of drug treatment for the year 2000 was estimated to be £69.5 million (including costs for anticoagulation clinic visits) and a further £271.6 million was spent on hospital admissions. These figures do not assume costs for hospitalisations where AF is a secondary diagnosis, or costs of nursing care.

A clinical need for the guideline is justified by the wide variation in management and disagreement amongst UK consultants regarding the best treatment strategies. Furthermore, many patients with AF possess very limited knowledge of AF, its consequences and therapy.

The guideline

The guideline development process is described in detail in two publications which are available from the NICE website (see further information section below). *The guideline development process – an overview for stakeholders, the public and the NHS*[15] describes how organisations can become involved in the development of a guideline. *Guideline development methods – information for national collaborating centres and guideline developers*[16] provides advice on the technical aspects of guideline development.

This document is the scope. It defines exactly what this guideline will (and will not) examine, and what the guideline developers will consider. The scope is based on the referral from the Department of Health and Welsh Assembly Government (see below).

The areas that will be addressed by the guideline are described in the following sections.

Population

▷ Groups that will be covered

The guideline will include people with:
- New onset or acute AF.
- Chronic AF, including paroxysmal (recurrent), persistent and permanent/sustained AF.
- Comorbidities that impact upon AF.
- Postoperative AF.
- Atrial flutter that is indistinguishable from AF in terms of aim of treatment.

▷ Groups that will not be covered

- People under age 18 years.
- Congenital heart disease precipitating AF.

Healthcare setting

Primary and secondary NHS healthcare settings, including referral to tertiary care.

Clinical management

Objectives of management are dependent upon clinical subtype of AF. AF is considered recurrent when a patient develops two or more episodes. These episodes may be paroxysmal if they terminate spontaneously (defined by consensus as 7 days), or persistent (usually more than 7 days) if the arrhythmia requires electrical or pharmacological cardioversion for termination. Successful termination of AF does not alter the classification of persistent AF in these patients. Longstanding AF (defined as more than 1 year) not successfully terminated by cardioversion, or when cardioversion is not pursued, is classified as permanent.

Treatment of acute, sudden onset of AF (with consideration of haemodynamic stability) will be distinguished from treatment of chronic (paroxysmal/recurrent, persistent and permanent) AF. Management of paroxysmal and persistent AF requires control of the rhythm, whilst in permanent AF; the management is generally rate control.

The guideline will include recommendations in the following areas.

▷ Identification of AF

The guideline will not cover general population screening but will include opportunistic case finding.

▷ Diagnosis and assessment criteria

The investigations required for accurate confirmation of a diagnosis of AF and assessment of comorbidity in AF including electrocardiogram (single and 12-lead), 24-hour ECG (or cardiomemo), echocardiogram (including transesophageal), chest X-ray and appropriate haematological and biochemical testing.

▷ Treatment

Treatment as defined for clinical subgroups of paroxysmal, persistent and permanent AF to include the following:

- Prophylactic antithrombotic treatment for the prevention of stroke and thromboembolism, to include antiplatelet and anticoagulation therapy as they specifically relate to AF, and take into account the following:
  - Risk stratification (for example low, medium and high risk) for thromboprophylaxis, including primary and secondary prevention.
  - Different populations (eg acute AF, and peri-stroke).
  - Use of anticoagulation in primary and secondary care setting as supported by the evidence. This includes the potential for management in primary care and self-management using near-patient testing devices.
- Rhythm control including pharmacological (oral and IV) and rhythm self-management ('pill-in-the-pocket') including maintenance of sinus rhythm post conversion.
- Pharmacological rate control (excluding non-pharmacological pacing and ablation, see below) pertaining to monotherapy and combination therapy.
- Efficacy of rate versus rhythm control.
- Selection of patients for referral to specialist services pertaining to non-pharmacological rhythm or rate control (pacing and catheter ablation) and electrophysiological studies.

▷ Review and monitoring

The review and monitoring of AF pertaining to the following:

- The benefits and harms of pharmacological and antithrombotic treatments (eg treatment side effects, and when to stop drug therapy).
- Maintenance of sinus rhythm.
- Patients in whom medical therapy has brought about no response.

Note that guideline recommendations will normally fall within licensed indications; exceptionally, and only where clearly supported by evidence, use outside a licensed indication may be recommended. The guideline will assume that prescribers will use the Summary of Product characteristics to inform their decisions for individual patients.

The following interventions/management will not be included in the guideline:
- Radical therapies that do not form common clinical management will not be addressed, including:
  - Implantable atrial defibrillator (IAD) as the evidence pertains to a selective group of patients and further clinical trials are required.
  - MAZE procedure and other arrhythmia surgery, as well as other novel/experimental non-pharmacological techniques (except for referral for these options).
  - Novel/experimental pharmaceutical antiarrhythmic agents.
- The impact of co-morbidities on AF will be considered but specific treatment of those comorbidities will not be included.
- Generic health problems where the care for people with AF disease does not differ from that of the general population (eg depression).

Status

This is the final scope, which has been through a 4-week period of consultation with stakeholders and has been reviewed by the Institute's independent Guidelines Review Panel.

NICE is in the process of developing the technology appraisal guidance. The AF guideline will signpost these technology appraisals and will consider their role in the treatment of AF.

Implantable cardioverter defibrillators (ICDs) for the treatment of arrhythmias – review of Guidance number 11. Expected date of publication July 2004

Stroke prevention: Ximelagatran in patients with stroke and other thromboembolic complications associated with fibrillation. Expected date of publication February 2006

The development of the guideline recommendations will begin in July 2004.

Further information

Information on the guideline development process is provided in:

The guideline development process – an overview for stakeholders, the public and the NHS[15]

Guideline development methods – information for national collaborating centres and guideline developers.[16]

These booklets are available as PDF files from the NICE website (**www.nice.org.uk**). Information on the progress of the guideline will also be available from the website.

Referral from the Department of Health and Welsh Assembly Government

The Department of Health and Welsh Assembly Government asked the Institute:

'To develop a guideline on the appropriate treatment of atril fibrillation (AF). This should include:

- Identification of patients with AF and appropriate risk assessment tools.
- Diagnosis and assessment.
- Appropriate treatment including:
    - antithrombotic treatment and appropriate use of antiplatelet and anti-coagulation therapy, including advice on potential for management in primary care and self-management using near patient testing devices
    - therapy to control rate of AF
    - medical and electrical cardioversion to control rhythm
    - selection of patients for referral to more specialist services, eg electrophysiological studies, pacing, catheter ablation and, if there is sufficient evidence, the role of ICDs.
- Review and monitoring of condition.'

References

1   Levy S, Camm AJ, Saksena S et al. International consensus on nomenclature and classification of atrial fibrillation; a collaborative project of the Working Group on Arrhythmias and the Working Group on Cardiac Pacing of the European Society of Cardiology and the North American Society of Pacing and Electrophysiology. *Europace*. 2003;5(2):119–122.

2   Lip GY, Golding DJ, Nazir M et al. A survey of atrial fibrillation in general practice: the West Birmingham Atrial Fibrillation Project. *British Journal of General Practice*. 1997;47(418):285–289.

3   Kannel WB, Wolf PA, Benjamin EJ et al. Prevalence, incidence, prognosis, and predisposing conditions for atrial fibrillation: population-based estimates. *American Journal of Cardiology*. 1998;82(8A):2N–9N.

4   Stewart S, Hart CL, Hole DJ et al. Population prevalence, incidence, and predictors of atrial fibrillation in the Renfrew/Paisley study. *Heart* (British Cardiac Society). 2001;86(5):516–521.

5   Lip GY, Bawden L, Hodson R et al. Atrial fibrillation amongst the Indo-Asian general practice population: the West Birmingham Atrial Fibrillation Project. *International Journal of Cardiology*. 1998;65(2):187–192.

6   Sudlow M, Thomson R, Thwaites B et al. Prevalence of atrial fibrillation and eligibility for anticoagulants in the community. *Lancet*. 1998;352(9135):1167–1171.

7   Lip GY, Tean KN, Dunn FG. Treatment of atrial fibrillation in a district general hospital. *British Heart Journal*. 1994;71(1):92–95.

8   Zarifis J, Beevers G, Lip GY. Acute admissions with atrial fibrillation in a British multiracial hospital population. *British Journal of Clinical Practice*. 1997;51(2):91–96.

9   Benjamin EJ, Levy D, Vaziri SM et al. Independent risk factors for atrial fibrillation in a population–based cohort. The Framingham Heart Study. *Journal of the American Medical Association*. 1994;271(11):840–844.

10 Lowenstein SR, Gabow PA, Cramer J et al. The role of alcohol in new–onset atrial fibrillation. *Archives of Internal Medicine*. 1983;143(10):1882–1885.

11 Benjamin EJ, Wolf PA, D'Agostino RB et al. Impact of atrial fibrillation on the risk of death: the Framingham Heart Study. *Circulation*. 1998;98(10):946–952.

12 Lip GY. Does atrial fibrillation confer a hypercoagulable state? *Lancet*. 1995;346(8986):1313–1314.

13 Wolf PA, Abbott RD, Kannel WB. Atrial fibrillation as an independent risk factor for stroke: the Framingham Study. *Stroke*. 1991;22(8):983–988.

14 Wolf PA, Mitchell JB, Baker CS et al. Impact of atrial fibrillation on mortality, stroke, and medical costs. *Archives of Internal Medicine*. 1998;158(3):229–234.

15 National Institute for Clinical Excellence. *The guideline development process – an overview for stakeholders, the public and the NHS*. London: National Institute for Clinical Excellence, 2005.

16 National Institute for Clinical Excellence. *Guideline development methods: information for national collaborating centres and guideline developers*. London: National Institute for Clinical Excellence, 2004.

17 National Collaborating Centre for Chronic Conditions. *NCC CC Methodology Pack*. London: NCC–CC;2005.

18 Freestone B, Lip G. Epidemiology and costs of cardiac arrhythmias. In: Lip G, Godtfredsen J (eds), *Cardiac Arrythmias: A clinical approach.*, Edinburgh: Mosby, 2003:3–24.

19 Swancutt D, Hobbs R, Fitzmaurice D et al. A randomised controlled trial and cost effectiveness study of systematic screening (targeted and total population screening) versus routine practice for the detection of atrial fibrillation in the over 65s. *BMC Cardiovascular Disorders*. 2004;4(1):12.

20 Hobbs FD, Fitzmaurice DA, Mant J et al. A randomised controlled trial and cost effectiveness study of systematic screening (targeted and total population screening) versus routine practice for the detection of atrial fibrillation in people aged 65 and over. The SAFE study. *Health Technology Assessment*. Winchester, 2005;9(40):1–90.

21 Davidson E, Rotenberg Z, Weinberger I et al. Diagnosis and characteristics of lone atrial fibrillation. *Chest*. 1989;95(5):1048–1050.

22 Lok N-S, Lau C-P. Presentation and management of patients admitted with atrial fibrillation: A review of 291 cases in a regional hospital. *International Journal of Cardiology*. 1995;48(3):271–278.

23 Shatoor AS, Ahmed ME, Said MA et al. Patterns of atrial fibrillation at a regional hospital in Saudi Arabia. *Ethnicity & Disease*. 1998;8(3):360–366.

24 Levy S, Maarek M, Coumel P et al. Characterization of different subsets of atrial fibrillation in general practice in France: the ALFA study. The College of French Cardiologists. *Circulation*. 1999;99(23):3028–3035.

25 Lin H, Wolf PA, Benjamin EJ et al. Newly diagnosed atrial fibrillation and acute stroke: the Framingham Study. *Stroke*. 1995;26(9):1527–1530.

26 Michael JA, Stiell IG, Agarwal S et al. Cardioversion of paroxysmal atrial fibrillation in the emergency department. *Annals of Emergency Medicine*. 1999;33(4):379–387.

27 Burton JH, Vinson DR, Drummond K et al. Electrical cardioversion of emergency department patients with atrial fibrillation. *Annals of Emergency Medicine*. 2004;44(1):20–30.

28 van Walraven C, Hart RG, Wells GA et al. A clinical prediction rule to identify patients with atrial fibrillation and a low risk for stroke while taking aspirin. *Archives of Internal Medicine*. 2003;163(8):936–943.

29 Sudlow M, Rodgers H, Kenny RA et al. Identification of patients with atrial fibrillation in general practice: a study of screening methods. *British Medical Journal*. 1998;317(7154):327–328.

30 Morgan S, Mant D. Randomised trial of two approaches to screening for atrial fibrillation in UK general practice. *British Journal of General Practice*. 2002;52(478):373–380.

31 Page RL, Wilkinson WE, Clair WK et al. Asymptomatic arrhythmias in patients with symptomatic paroxysmal atrial fibrillation and paroxysmal supraventricular tachycardia. *Circulation*. 1994;89(1):224–227.

32 Kinlay S, Leitch JW, Neil A et al. Cardiac event recorders yield more diagnoses and are more cost-effective than 48-hour Holter monitoring in patients with palpitations: a controlled clinical trial. *Annals of Internal Medicine*. 1996;124(1 Pt 1):16–20.

33 Reiffel JA, Schwarzberg R, Murry M. Comparison of autotriggered memory loop recorders versus standard loop recorders versus 24-hour Holter monitors for arrhythmia detection. *American Journal of Cardiology*. 2005;95(9):1055–1059.

34 Man-Son-Hing M, Laupacis A. Anticoagulant-related bleeding in older persons with atrial fibrillation: physicians' fears often unfounded. *Archives of Internal Medicine*. 2003;163(13):1580–1586.

35 Jabaudon D, Sztajzel J, Sievert K et al. Usefulness of ambulatory 7-day ECG monitoring for the detection of atrial fibrillation and flutter after acute stroke and transient ischemic attack. *Stroke*. 2004;35(7):1647–1651.

36 Lip G, Zarifis J, Watson R et al. Physician variation in the management of patients with atrial fibrillation. *Heart* (British Cardiac Society) 1996;75(2):200–205.

37 Lip GY. How would I manage a 60-year-old woman presenting with atrial fibrillation? *Proceedings of the Royal College of Physicians of Edinburgh*. 2005;1999(29):301–306.

38 Cantley P, McKinstry B, Macaulay D et al. Atrial fibrillation in general practice: how useful is echo-cardiography in selection of suitable patients for anticoagulation? *British Journal of General Practice*. 1999;49(440):219–220.

39 Klein AL, Murray RD, Grimm RA. Role of transesophageal echocardiography-guided cardioversion of patients with atrial fibrillation. *Journal of the American College of Cardiology*. 2001;37(3):691–704.

40 Flaker GC, Fletcher KA, Rothbart RM et al. Clinical and echocardiographic features of intermittent atrial fibrillation that predict recurrent atrial fibrillation. *American Journal of Cardiology*. 1995;76(5):355–358.

41 Tischler MD, Lee TH, McAndrew KA et al. Clinical, echocardiographic and Doppler correlates of clinical instability with onset of atrial fibrillation. *American Journal of Cardiology*. 1990;66(7):721–724.

42 Antonielli E, Pizzuti A, Palinkas A et al. Clinical value of left atrial appendage flow for prediction of long-term sinus rhythm maintenance in patients with nonvalvular atrial fibrillation. *Journal of the American College of Cardiology*. 2002;39(9):1443–1449.

43 Roijer A, Meurling CJ, Eskilsson J et al. Left atrial appendage outflow velocity index is superior to conventional criteria for prediction of maintenance of sinus rhythm after cardioversion. *Scandinavian Cardiovascular Journal.* 2001;35(2):119–124.

44 Dogan A, Avsar A, Ozturk M. P-wave dispersion for predicting maintenance of sinus rhythm after cardioversion of atrial fibrillation. *American Journal of Cardiology.* 2004;93(3):368–371.

45 Frick M, Frykman V, Jensen-Urstad M et al. Factors predicting success rate and recurrence of atrial fibrillation after first electrical cardioversion in patients with persistent atrial fibrillation. *Clinical Cardiology.* 2001;24(3):238–244.

46 Duytschaever M, Haerynck F, Tavernier R et al. Factors influencing long-term persistence of sinus rhythm after a first electrical cardioversion for atrial fibrillation. *Pacing and Clinical Electrophysiology.* 1998;21(1 II SUPPL.):284–287.

47 Arnar DO, Danielsen R. Factors predicting maintenance of sinus rhythm after direct current cardioversion of atrial fibrillation and flutter: a reanalysis with recently acquired data. *Cardiology.* 1996;87(3):181–188.

48 Olshansky B, Heller EN, Mitchell LB et al. Are transthoracic echocardiographic parameters associated with atrial fibrillation recurrence or stroke? Results from the Atrial Fibrillation Follow-Up Investigation of Rhythm Management (AFFIRM) study. *Journal of the American College of Cardiology.* 2005;45(12): 2026–2033.

49 Dmochowska-Perz M, Loboz-Grudzien K, Sokalski L et al. Factors predicting recurrence of atrial fibrillation after cardioversion. *Kardiologia Polska.* 2002;57(12):501–511.

50 Paraskevaidis IA, Dodouras T, Tsiapras D et al. Prediction of successful cardioversion and maintenance of sinus rhythm in patients with lone atrial fibrillation. *Chest.* 2005;127(2):488–494.

51 Leung DY, Black IW, Cranney GB et al. Prognostic implications of left atrial spontaneous echo contrast in nonvalvular atrial fibrillation. *Journal of the American College of Cardiology.* 1994;24(3):755–762.

52 Aronow WS, Gutstein H, Hsieh FY. Risk factors for thromboembolic stroke in elderly patients with chronic atrial fibrillation. *American Journal of Cardiology.* 1989;63(5):366–367.

53 Shinokawa N, Hirai T, Takashima S et al. A transesophageal echocardiographic study on risk factors for stroke in elderly patients with atrial fibrillation: a comparison with younger patients. *Chest.* 2001;120(3): 840–846.

54 Stollberger C, Chnupa P, Kronik G et al. Transesophageal echocardiography to assess embolic risk in patients with atrial fibrillation. ELAT study group: embolism in left atrial thrombi. *Annals of Internal Medicine.* 1998;128(8):630–638.

55 Miyazaki S, Ito T, Suwa M et al. Role of transesophageal echocardiography in the prediction of thromboembolism in patients with chronic nonvalvular atrial fibrillation. *Japanese Circulation Journal.* 2001; 65(10):874–878.

56 Kamp O, Verhorst PMJ, Welling RC et al. Importance of left atrial appendage flow as a predictor of thromboembolic events in patients with atrial fibrillation. *European Heart Journal.* 1999;20(13):979–985.

57 Pearce LA. Predictors of thromboembolism in atrial fibrillation (II): echocardiographic features of patients at risk. *Annals of Internal Medicine.* 1992;116(1):6–12.

58 Kosior D, Szulc M, Piatkowski R et al. Factors determining long-term maintenance of sinus rhythm after cardioversion of persistent atrial fibrillation. *Kardiologia Polska.* 2003;59:128 141.

59 Nakagami H, Yamamoto K, Ikeda U et al. Mitral regurgitation reduces the risk of stroke in patients with nonrheumatic atrial fibrillation. *American Heart Journal.* 1998;136(3):528–532.

60 Cabin HS, Clubb KS, Hall C et al. Risk for systemic embolization of atrial fibrillation without mitral stenosis. *American Journal of Cardiology.* 1990;65(16):1112–1116.

61 Ezekowitz MD, Laupacis A, Boysen G et al. Echocardiographic predictors of stroke in patients with atrial fibrillation: a prospective study of 1,066 patients from 3 clinical trials. *Archives of Internal Medicine.* 1998;158(12):1316–1320.

62 Aronow WS, Ahn C, Kronzon I et al. Risk factors for new thromboembolic stroke in patients <=62 years of age with chronic atrial fibrillation. *American Journal of Cardiology.* 1998;82(1):119–121.

63   Dawn B, Varma J, Singh P et al. Cardiovascular death in patients with atrial fibrillation is better predicted by left atrial thrombus and spontaneous echocardiographic contrast as compared with clinical parameters. *Journal of the American Society of Echocardiography.* 2005;18(3):199–205.

64   Conway D. Cardioversion of persistent atrial fibrillation. In: Lip GY, Godfredsen J (eds), *Cardiac arrhythmias: a clinical approach,* Edinburgh: Mosby, 2003: 299–318.

65   Lim H, Hamaad A, Lip G. Clinical review: clinical management of atrial fibrillation – rate control versus rhythm control. *Critical Care.* 8(4);271–279. 2004.

66   Rashba EJ, Gold MR, Crawford FA et al. Efficacy of transthoracic cardioversion of atrial fibrillation using a biphasic, truncated exponential shock waveform at variable initial shock energies. *American Journal of Cardiology.* 2004;94(12):1572–1574.

67   Adgey AA, Walsh SJ. Theory and practice of defibrillation: (1) atrial fibrillation and DC conversion. *Heart.* 2004;90(12):1493–1498.

68   Lip GY. Cardioversion of atrial fibrillation. *Postgraduate Medical Journal.* 1995;71(838):457–465.

69   de Paola AA, Figueiredo E, Sesso R et al. Effectiveness and costs of chemical versus electrical cardioversion of atrial fibrillation. *International Journal of Cardiology.* 2003;88(2–3):157–3.

70   Valencia MJ, Climent P, V, Marin O et al. The efficacy of scheduled cardioversion in atrial fibrillation: comparison of two schemes of treatment: electrical versus pharmacological cardioversion. *Revista Espanola de Cardiologia.* 2002;55(22–3):113–120.

71   Boodhoo L, Bordoli G, Mitchell AR et al. The safety and effectiveness of a nurse-led cardioversion service under sedation. *Heart.* 2004;90(12):1443–1446.

72   Currie MP, Karwatowski SP, Perera J et al. Introduction of nurse led DC cardioversion service in day surgery unit: Prospective audit. *British Medical Journal.* 2004;329(7471):892–894.

73   Quinn T. Early experience of nurse-led elective DC cardioversion. *Nursing in Critical Care.* 1998;3(2):59–62.

74   Naccarelli GV, Wolbrette DL, Luck JC. Proarrhythmia. *Medical Clinics of North America.* 2001;85(2): 503–526.

75   Chaudhry GM, Haffajee CI. Antiarrhythmic agents and proarrhythmia. *Critical Care Medicine.* 2000; 28(10 Suppl):N158–N164.

76   Podrid PJ. Proarrhythmia, a serious complication of antiarrhythmic drugs. *Current Cardiology Reports.* 1999;1(4):289–296.

77   Mooss AN, Wurdeman RL, Mohiuddin SM et al. Esmolol versus diltiazem in the treatment of postoperative atrial fibrillation/atrial flutter after open heart surgery. *American Heart Journal.* 2000;140(1): 176–180.

78   Hilleman DE, Reyes AP, Mooss AN et al. Esmolol versus diltiazem in atrial fibrillation following coronary artery bypass graft surgery. *Current Medical Research & Opinion.* 2003;19(5):376–382.

79   Anon. Intravenous digoxin in acute atrial fibrillation: results of a randomized, placebo-controlled multicentre trial in 239 patients. The Digitalis in Acute Atrial Fibrillation (DAAF) Trial Group. *European Heart Journal.* 1997;18(4):649–654.

80   Jordaens L, Trouerbach J, Calle P et al. Conversion of atrial fibrillation to sinus rhythm and rate control by digoxin in comparison to placebo. *European Heart Journal.* 1997;18(4):643–648.

81   Falk RH, Knowlton AA, Bernard SA et al. Digoxin for converting recent–onset atrial fibrillation to sinus rhythm. A randomized, double-blinded trial. *Annals of Internal Medicine.* 1987;106(4):503–506.

82   Andrivet P, Boubakri E, Dove PJ et al. A clinical study of amiodarone as a single oral dose in patients with recent-onset atrial tachyarrhythmia. *European Heart Journal.* 1994;15(10):1396–1402.

83   Boriani G, Capucci A, Lenzi T et al. Propafenone for conversion of recent–onset atrial fibrillation. A controlled comparison between oral loading dose and intravenous administration. *Chest.* 1995;108(2): 355–358.

84   Botto GL, Bonini W, Broffoni T et al. Randomized, crossover, controlled comparison of oral loading versus intravenous infusion of propafenone in recent-onset atrial fibrillation. *Pacing and Clinical Electrophysiology.* 1998;21(11 Pt 2):2480–2484.

85 Boriani G, Biffi M, Capucci A et al. Conversion of recent-onset atrial fibrillation to sinus rhythm: effects of different drug protocols. *Pacing and Clinical Electrophysiology.* 1998;21(11 Pt 2):2470–2474.

86 Chevalier P, Durand–Dubief A, Burri H et al. Amiodarone versus placebo and classic drugs for cardioversion of recent-onset atrial fibrillation: a meta-analysis. *Journal of the American College of Cardiology.* 2003;41(2):255–262.

87 Treglia A, Alfano C, Rossini E. A comparison between propafenone and amiodarone in the conversion to sinus rhythm of atrial fibrillation of recent onset. *Minerva Cardioangiologica.* 1994;42(6):293–297.

88 Joseph AP, Ward MR. A prospective, randomized controlled trial comparing the efficacy and safety of sotalol, amiodarone, and digoxin for the reversion of new-onset atrial fibrillation. *Annals of Emergency Medicine.* 2000;36(1):1–9.

89 Singh BN, Singh SN, Reda DJ et al. Amiodarone versus sotalol for atrial fibrillation. *New England Journal of Medicine.* 2005;352(18):1861–1872.

90 Martinez–Marcos FJ, Garcia-Garmendia JL, Ortega-Carpio A et al. Comparison of intravenous flecainide, propafenone, and amiodarone for conversion of acute atrial fibrillation to sinus rhythm. *American Journal of Cardiology.* 2000;86(9):950–953.

91 Kochiadakis GE, Igoumenidis NE, Simantirakis EN et al. Intravenous propafenone versus intravenous amiodarone in the management of atrial fibrillation of recent onset: a placebo-controlled study. *Pacing and Clinical Electrophysiology.* 1998;21(11 Pt 2):2475–2479.

92 Donovan KD, Power BM, Hockings BE et al. Intravenous flecainide versus amiodarone for recent-onset atrial fibrillation. *American Journal of Cardiology.* 1995;75(10):693–697.

93 Negrini M, Gibelli G, De Ponti C. A comparison of propafenone and amiodarone in reversion of recent-onset atrial fibrillation to sinus rhythm. *Current Therapeutic Research, Clinical & Experimental.* 1994; 55(11):1345–1354.

94 Blanc JJ, Voinov C, Maarek M. Comparison of oral loading dose of propafenone and amiodarone for converting recent-onset atrial fibrillation. PARSIFAL study group. *American Journal of Cardiology.* 1999;84(9):1029–1032.

95 Baldi N, Lenti V, Marasco G et al. Propafenone vs flecainide in the acute treatment of atrial fibrillation of recent onset: a randomized study. *New Trends in Arrhythmias.* 1992;8(1–2):499–505.

96 Kondili A, Kastrati A, Popa Y. Comparative evaluation of verapamil, flecainide and propafenone for the acute conversion of atrial fibrillation to sinus rhythm. *Middle European Journal of Medicine.* 1990;102(17): 510–513.

97 Kingma JH, Suttorp MJ. Acute pharmacologic conversion of atrial fibrillation and flutter: the role of flecainide, propafenone, and verapamil. *American Journal of Cardiology.* 1992;70(5):56A–60A.

98 Capucci A, Boriani G, Botto GL et al. Conversion of recent-onset atrial fibrillation by a single oral loading dose of propafenone or flecainide. *American Journal of Cardiology.* 1994;74(5):503–505.

99 Van Gelder IC, Tuinenburg AE, Schoonderwoerd BS et al. Pharmacologic versus direct-current electrical cardioversion of atrial flutter and fibrillation. *American Journal of Cardiology.* 1999;84(9A):147R–151R.

100 Climent VE, Marin F, Mainar L et al. Effects of pretreatment with intravenous flecainide on efficacy of external cardioversion of persistent atrial fibrillation. *Pacing and Clinical Electrophysiology.* 2004;27(3):368–372.

101 Channer KS, Birchall A, Steeds RP et al. A randomized placebo-controlled trial of pre-treatment and short- or long-term maintenance therapy with amiodarone supporting DC cardioversion for persistent atrial fibrillation. *European Heart Journal.* 2004;25(2):144–150.

102 Bianconi L, Mennuni M, Lukic V et al. Pretreatment with oral propafenone in electrical cardioversion of chronic atrial fibrillation. *New Trends in Arrhythmias.* 1993;9(4):1017–1020.

103 Bianconi L, Mennuni M, Lukic V et al. Effects of oral propafenone administration before electrical cardioversion of chronic atrial fibrillation: a placebo-controlled study. *Journal of the American College of Cardiology.* 1996;28(3):700–706.

104 Jacobs LO, Andrews TC, Pederson DN et al. Effect of intravenous procainamide on direct-current cardioversion of atrial fibrillation. *American Journal of Cardiology.* 1998;82(2):241–242.

105 Villani GQ, Piepoli MF, Terracciano C et al. Effects of diltiazem pretreatment on direct-current cardioversion in patients with persistent atrial fibrillation: A single-blind, randomized, controlled study. *American Heart Journal.* 2000;140:437–443.

106 Jong G-P, Hou Z-Y, Juang G-H et al. Short term amiodarone treatment facilitates electrical cardioversion in patients with chronic atrial flutter/fibrillation. *Acta Cardiologica Sinica.* 1995;11(1):39–46.

107 Capucci A, Villani GQ, Aschieri D et al. Oral amiodarone increases the efficacy of direct-current cardioversion in restoration of sinus rhythm in patients with chronic atrial fibrillation. *European Heart Journal.* 2000;21(1):66–73.

108 Lindholm C-J, Fredholm O, Moller S-J et al. Sinus rhythm maintenance following DC cardioversion of atrial fibrillation is not improved by temporary pre-cardioversion treatment with oral verapamil. *Heart* (British Cardiac Society), 2004;90(5):534–538.

109 De Simone A, Stabile G, Vitale DF et al. Pretreatment with verapamil in patients with persistent or chronic atrial fibrillation who underwent electrical cardioversion. *Journal of the American College of Cardiology.* 1999;34(3):810–814.

110 Bertaglia E, D'Este D, Zanocco A et al. Effects of pretreatment with verapamil on early recurrences after electrical cardioversion of persistent atrial fibrillation: a randomised study. *Heart.* 2001;85:578–580.

111 AFFIRM First-Antiarrhythmic-Drug-Substudy-Investigators. Maintenance of sinus rhythm in patients with atrial fibrillation: an AFFIRM substudy of the first antiarrhythmic drug. *Journal of the American College of Cardiology.* 2003;42(1):20–29.

112 Roy D, Talajic M, Dorian P et al. Amiodarone to prevent recurrence of atrial fibrillation: Canadian Trial of Atrial Fibrillation Investigators. *New England Journal of Medicine.* 2000;342(13):913–920.

113 Guo H, Shaheen W, Kerber R et al. Cardioversion of atrial tachyarrhythmias: anticoagulation to reduce thromboembolic complications. *Progress in Cardiovascular Diseases.* 2004;46(6):487–505.

114 Klein AL, Grimm RA, Murray RD et al. Use of transesophageal echocardiography to guide cardioversion in patients with atrial fibrillation. *New England Journal of Medicine.* 2001;344(19):1411–1420.

115 Seidl K, Rameken M, Drogemuller A et al. Embolic events in patients with atrial fibrillation and effective anticoagulation: value of transesophageal echocardiography to guide direct-current cardioversion. Final results of the Ludwigshafen Observational Cardioversion Study. *Journal of the American College of Cardiology.* 2002;39(9):1436–1442.

116 Klein AL, Murray RD, Becker ER et al. Economic analysis of a transesophageal echocardiography-guided approach to cardioversion of patients with atrial fibrillation: the ACUTE economic data at eight weeks. *Journal of the American College of Cardiology.* 2004;43(7):1217–1224.

117 Seto TB, Taira DA, Tsevat J et al. Cost-effectiveness of transesophageal echocardiographic-guided cardioversion: a decision analytic model for patients admitted to the hospital with atrial fibrillation. *Journal of the American College of Cardiology.* 1997;29(1):122–130.

118 Van Gelder IC, Hagens VE, Bosker HA et al. A comparison of rate control and rhythm control in patients with recurrent persistent atrial fibrillation. *New England Journal of Medicine.* 2002;347(23):1834–1840.

119 Carlsson J, Miketic S, Windeler J et al. Randomized trial of rate-control versus rhythm-control in persistent atrial fibrillation: the Strategies of Treatment of Atrial Fibrillation (STAF) Study. *Journal of the American College of Cardiology.* 2003;41(10):1690–1696.

120 Gronefeld GC, Lilienthal J, Kuck KH et al. Impact of rate versus rhythm control on quality of life in patients with persistent atrial fibrillation. Results from a prospective randomized study. *European Heart Journal.* 2003;24:1430–1436.

121 Wyse DG, Waldo AL, DiMarco JP et al. A comparison of rate control and rhythm control in patients with atrial fibrillation. *New England Journal of Medicine.* 2002;347:1825–1833.

122 Opolski G, Torbicki A, Kosior D et al. Rhythm control versus rate control in patients with persistent atrial fibrillation. Results of the HOT CAFE Polish Study. *Kardiologia Polska.* 2003;59(7):1–16.

123 Hagens VE, Crijns HJ, Van Veldhuisen DJ et al. Rate control versus rhythm control for patients with persistent atrial fibrillation with mild to moderate heart failure: results from the RAte Control versus Electrical cardioversion (RACE) study. *American Heart Journal.* 2005;149(6):1106–1111.

124   de Denus S, Sanoski CA, Carlsson J et al. Rate vs rhythm control in patients with atrial fibrillation: a meta-analysis. *Archives of Internal Medicine.* 2005;165(3):258–262.

125   Marshall DA, Levy AR, Vidaillet H et al. Cost-effectiveness of rhythm versus rate control in atrial fibrillation. *Annals of Internal Medicine.* 2004;141(9):653–661.

126   Hagens VE, Vermeulen KM, TenVergert EM et al. Rate control is more cost-effective than rhythm control for patients with persistent atrial fibrillation – results from the RAte Control versus Electrical cardioversion (RACE) study. *European Heart Journal.* 2004;25(17):1542–1549.

127   Corley SD, Epstein AE, DiMarco JP et al. Relationships between sinus rhythm, treatment, and survival in the Atrial Fibrillation Follow-Up Investigation of Rhythm Management (AFFIRM) Study. *Circulation.* 2004;109(12):1509–1513.

128   McNamara RL, Tamariz LJ, Segal JB et al. Management of atrial fibrillation: review of the evidence for the role of pharmacologic therapy, electrical cardioversion, and echocardiography. *Annals of Internal Medicine.* 2003;139(12):1018–1033.

129   Coplen SE, Antman EM, Berlin JA et al. Efficacy and safety of quinidine therapy for maintenance of sinus rhythm after cardioversion. A meta-analysis of randomized control trials (erratum appears in *Circulation* 1991;83(2):714). *Circulation.* 1990;82(4):1106–1116.

130   De Simone A, De Pasquale M, De Matteis C et al. Verapamil plus antiarrhythmic drugs reduce atrial fibrillation recurrences after an electrical cardioversion (VEPARAF study). *European Heart Journal.* 2003;24(15):1425–1429.

131   Kochiadakis GE, Igoumenidis NE, Marketou ME et al. Low-dose amiodarone versus sotalol for suppression of recurrent symptomatic atrial fibrillation. *American Journal of Cardiology.* 1998;81(8): 995–998.

132   Kochiadakis GE, Igoumenidis NE, Marketou ME et al. Low dose amiodarone and sotalol in the treatment of recurrent, symptomatic atrial fibrillation: a comparative, placebo-controlled study. *Heart.* 2000;84(3): 251–257.

133   Kochiadakis GE, Marketou ME, Igoumenidis NE et al. Amiodarone, sotalol, or propafenone in atrial fibrillation: which is preferred to maintain normal sinus rhythm? *Pacing and Clinical Electrophysiology.* 2000;23(11 Pt 2):1883–1887.

134   Bellandi F, Simonetti I, Leoncini M et al. Long-term efficacy and safety of propafenone and sotalol for the maintenance of sinus rhythm after conversion of recurrent symptomatic atrial fibrillation. *American Journal of Cardiology.* 2001;88(6):640–645.

135   Reimold SC, Cantillon CO, Friedman PL et al. Propafenone vs sotalol for suppression of recurrent symptomatic atrial fibrillation. *American Journal of Cardiology.* 1993;71(7):558–563.

136   Kochiadakis GE, Igoumenidis NE, Hamilos ME et al. Sotalol vs propafenone for long-term maintenance of normal sinus rhythm in patients with recurrent symptomatic atrial fibrillation. *American Journal of Cardiology.* 2004;94(12):1563–1566.

137   Kochiadakis GE, Igoumenidis NE, Hamilos MI et al. Long-term maintenance of normal sinus rhythm in patients with current symptomatic atrial fibrillation: amiodarone vs propafenone, both in low doses. *Chest.* 2004;125(2):377–383.

138   Plewan A, Lehmann G, Ndrepepa G et al. Maintenance of sinus rhythm after electrical cardioversion of persistent atrial fibrillation; sotalol versus bisoprolol. *European Heart Journal.* 2001;22(16):1504–1510.

139   Bjerkelund CJ, Orning OM. The efficacy of anticoagulant therapy in preventing embolism related to DC electrical conversion of atrial fibrillation. *American Journal of Cardiology.* 1969;23(2):208–216.

140   Weigner MJ, Caulfield TA, Danias PG et al. Risk for clinical thromboembolism associated with conversion to sinus rhythm in patients with atrial fibrillation lasting less than 48 hours. *Annals of Internal Medicine.* 1997;126(8):615–620.

141   Moreyra E, Finkelhor RS, Cebul RD. Limitations of transesophageal echocardiography in the risk assessment of patients before nonanticoagulated cardioversion from atrial fibrillation and flutter: an analysis of pooled trials. *American Heart Journal.* 1995;129(1):71–75.

142 Gentile F, Elhendy A, Khandheria BK et al. Safety of electrical cardioversion in patients with atrial fibrillation. *Mayo Clinic Proceedings.* 2002;77(9):897–904.

143 Gallagher MM, Hennessy BJ, Edvardsson N et al. Embolic complications of direct current cardioversion of atrial arrhythmias: association with low intensity of anticoagulation at the time of cardioversion. *Journal of the American College of Cardiology.* 2002;40(5):926–933.

144 Stellbrink C, Nixdorff U, Hofmann T et al. Safety and efficacy of enoxaparin compared with unfractionated heparin and oral anticoagulants for prevention of thromboembolic complications in cardioversion of nonvalvular atrial fibrillation: the Anticoagulation in Cardioversion using Enoxaparin (ACE) trial. *Circulation.* 2004;109(8):997–1003.

145 Collins LJ, Silverman DI, Douglas PS et al. Cardioversion of nonrheumatic atrial fibrillation. Reduced thromboembolic complications with 4 weeks of precardioversion anticoagulation are related to atrial thrombus resolution. *Circulation.* 1995;92(2):160–163.

146 Umana E, Solares CA, Alpert MA. Tachycardia-induced cardiomyopathy. *American Journal of Medicine.* 2003;114(1):51–55.

147 Royal College of Physicians of Edinburgh. Consensus Conference on Atrial Fibrillation: final consensus statement. Proceedings of the Royal College of Physicians of Edinburgh. 1998;28:552–4.

148 Falk RH, Leavitt J. Digoxin for atrial fibrillation: a drug whose time has gone? *Ann Intern Med.* 1991;114:573–75.

149 Li-Saw-Hee FL, Lip GY. Digoxin Revisted. *Quarterly Journal of Medicine.* 1998;91:259–264.

150 Freestone B, Lip GY. Heart rate control. In: Lip GYH, Godtfredsen J (eds), *Cardiac Arrhythmias: a clinical approach.* Edinburgh: Mosby, 2003:275–298.

151 Khand AU, Rankin AC, Martin W et al. Carvedilol alone or in combination with digoxin for the management of atrial fibrillation in patients with heart failure? *Journal of the American College of Cardiology.* 2003;42(11):1944–1951.

152 Koh KK, Song JH, Kwon KS et al. Comparative study of efficacy and safety of low-dose diltiazem or betaxolol in combination with digoxin to control ventricular rate in chronic atrial fibrillation: randomized crossover study. *International Journal of Cardiology.* 1995;52(2):167–174.

153 Lewis RV, McMurray J, McDevitt DG. Effects of atenolol, verapamil, and xamoterol on heart rate and exercise tolerance in digitalised patients with chronic atrial fibrillation. *Journal of Cardiovascular Pharmacology.* 1989;13(1):1–6.

154 Farshi R, Kistner D, Sarma JS et al. Ventricular rate control in chronic atrial fibrillation during daily activity and programmed exercise: a crossover open-label study of five drug regimens. *Journal of the American College of Cardiology.* 1999;33(2):304–310.

155 Maragno I, Santostasi G, Gaion RM et al. Low- and medium-dose diltiazem in chronic atrial fibrillation: comparison with digoxin and correlation with drug plasma levels. *American Heart Journal.* 1988;116(2 Pt 1):385–392.

156 Lewis RV, Laing E, Moreland TA et al. A comparison of digoxin, diltiazem and their combination in the treatment of atrial fibrillation. *European Heart Journal.* 1988;9(3):279–283.

157 Pomfret SM, Beasley CR, Challenor V et al. Relative efficacy of oral verapamil and digoxin alone and in combination for the treatment of patients with chronic atrial fibrillation. *Clinical Science.* 1988;74(4):351–357.

158 Lewis R, Lakhani M, Moreland TA et al. A comparison of verapamil and digoxin in the treatment of atrial fibrillation. *European Heart Journal.* 1987;8(2):148–153.

159 Roth A, Harrison E, Mitani G et al. Efficacy and safety of medium- and high-dose diltiazem alone and in combination with digoxin for control of heart-rate at rest and during exercise in patients with chronic atrial fibrillation. *Circulation.* 1986;73(2):316–324.

160 Botto GL, Bonini W, Broffoni T. Modulation of ventricular rate in permanent atrial fibrillation: randomized, crossover study of the effects of slow-release formulations of gallopamil, diltiazem, or verapamil. *Clinical Cardiology.* 1998;21(11):837–840.

161 Wong CK, Lau CP, Leung WH et al. Usefulness of labetalol in chronic atrial fibrillation. *American Journal of Cardiology.* 1990;66(17):1212–1215.

162 Lang R, Klein HO, Weiss E et al. Superiority of oral verapamil therapy to digoxin in treatment of chronic atrial fibrillation. *Chest.* 1983;83(3):491–499.

163 Fleming HA, Bailey SM. Mitral valve disease, systemic embolism and anticoagulants. *Postgraduate Medical Journal.* 1971;47(551):599–604.

164 Salem DN, Stein PD, Al Ahmad A et al. Antithrombotic therapy in valvular heart disease – native and prosthetic: the Seventh ACCP Conference on Antithrombotic and Thrombolytic Therapy. *Chest.* 2004;126(3 Suppl):457S–482S.

165 Szekely P. Systemic embolization and anticoagulant prophylaxis in rhuematic heart disease. *British Medical Journal.* 1964;1964(1):209–212.

166 Petersen P, Madsen EB, Brun B et al. Silent cerebral infarction in chronic atrial fibrillation. *Stroke.* 1987;18(6):1098–1100.

167 Wolf PA, Kannel WB, McGee DL et al. Duration of atrial fibrillation and imminence of stroke: the Framingham Study. *Stroke.* 1983;14(5):664–667.

168 Laupacis A, Boysen G, Connolly S et al. Risk factors for stroke and efficacy of antithrombotic therapy in atrial fibrillation: analysis of pooled data from five randomized controlled trials. *Archives of Internal Medicine.* 1994;154(13):1449–1457.

169 Lane D, Lip GY. Anti-thrombotic therapy for atrial fibrillation and patients' preferences for treatment. *Age & Ageing.* 2005;34(1):1–3.

170 Howitt A, Armstrong D. Implementing evidence based medicine in general practice: audit and qualitative study of antithrombotic treatment for atrial fibrillation. *British Medical Journal.* 1999;318(7194): 1324–1327.

171 Hart RG, Benavente O, McBride R et al. Antithrombotic therapy to prevent stroke in patients with atrial fibrillation: a meta-analysis. *Annals of Internal Medicine.* 1999;131(7):492–501.

172 Segal JB, McNamara RL, Miller MR et al. Anticoagulants or antiplatelet therapy for non-rheumatic atrial fibrillation and flutter. *The Cochrane Library.* 2004;(1)

173 Benavente O, Hart R, Koudstaal P et al. Oral anticoagulants for preventing stroke in patients with non-valvular atrial fibrillation and no previous history of stroke or transient ischemic attacks. *The Cochrane Library.* 2003;(4)

174 van Walraven C, Hart RG, Singer DE et al. Oral anticoagulants vs aspirin in nonvalvular atrial fibrillation: an individual patient meta-analysis. *Journal of the American Medical Association.* 2002;288(19):2441–2448.

175 Taylor FC, Cohen H, Ebrahim S. Systematic review of long-term anticoagulation or antiplatelet treatment in patients with non-rheumatic atrial fibrillation (erratum appears in BMJ 2001 Mar 10;322(7286):587). *British Medical Journal.* 2001;322(7282):321–326.

176 Hylek EM, Go AS, Chang Y et al. Effect of intensity of oral anticoagulation on stroke severity and mortality in atrial fibrillation. *New England Journal of Medicine.* 2003;349(11):1019–1026.

177 Perret-Guillaume C, Wahl DG. Low-dose warfarin in atrial fibrillation leads to more thromboembolic events without reducing major bleeding when compared to adjusted-dose. *Thrombosis & Haemostasis.* 2004;91(2):394–402.

178 Benavente O, Hart R, Koudstaal P et al. Antiplatelet therapy for preventing stroke in patients with non-valvular atrial fibrillation and no previous history of stroke or transient ischemic attacks. *The Cochrane Library.* 2003;(4)

179 Perez-Gomez F, Alegria E, Berjon J et al. Comparative effects of antiplatelet, anticoagulant, or combined therapy in patients with valvular and nonvalvular atrial fibrillation: a randomized multicenter study. *Journal of the American College of Cardiology.* 2004;44(8):1557–1566.

180 Lip GY, Kamath S, Jafri M et al. Ethnic differences in patient perceptions of atrial fibrillation and anticoagulation therapy: the West Birmingham Atrial Fibrillation Project. *Stroke.* 2002;33(1):238–242.

181   Antithrombotic TC. Collaborative meta-analysis of randomised trials of antiplatelet therapy for prevention of death, myocardial infarction, and stroke in high risk patients (erratum appears in *BMJ* 2002 Jan 19;324(7330):141). *British Medical Journal.* 2002;324(7329):71–86.

182   Petersen P, Boysen G, Godtfredsen J et al. Placebo-controlled, randomised trial of warfarin and aspirin for prevention of thromboembolic complications in chronic atrial fibrillation: the Copenhagen AFASK study. *Lancet.* 1989;1:175–179.

183   Singer DE, Hughes RA, Gress DR et al. The effect of aspirin on the risk of stroke in patients with nonrheumatic atrial fibrillation: the BAATAF Study. *American Heart Journal.* 1992;124(6):1567–1573.

184   McBride R. Stroke prevention in atrial fibrillation study: final results. *Circulation.* 1991;84(2):527–539.

185   Lip GYH, Li-Saw-Hee FL. Paroxysmal atrial fibrillation. *Quarterly Journal of Medicine.* 2001;94(12): 665–678.

186   Murgatroyd FD, Gibson SM, Baiyan X et al. Double-blind placebo-controlled trial of digoxin in symptomatic paroxysmal atrial fibrillation. *Circulation.* 1999;99(21):2765–2770.

187   Lee SH, Chen SA, Tai CT et al. Comparisons of oral propafenone and sotalol as an initial treatment in patients with symptomatic paroxysmal atrial fibrillation. *American Journal of Cardiology.* 1997;79(7): 905–908.

188   Steeds RP, Birchall AS, Smith M et al. An open label, randomised, crossover study comparing sotalol and atenolol in the treatment of symptomatic paroxysmal atrial fibrillation. *Heart.* 1999;82(2):170–175.

189   Lumer GB, Roy D, Talajic M et al. Amiodarone reduces procedures and costs related to atrial fibrillation in a controlled clinical trial. *European Heart Journal.* 2002;23(13):1050–1056.

190   Alboni P, Botto GL, Baldi N et al. Outpatient treatment of recent-onset atrial fibrillation with the 'pill-in-the-pocket' approach. *New England Journal of Medicine.* 2004;351(23):2384–2391.

191   Alboni P, Tomasi C, Menozzi C et al. Efficacy and safety of out-of-hospital self-administered single-dose oral drug treatment in the management of infrequent, well-tolerated paroxysmal supraventricular tachycardia. *Journal of the American College of Cardiology.* 2001;37(2):548–553.

192   Hart RG, Pearce LA, Rothbart RM et al. Stroke with intermittent atrial fibrillation: incidence and predictors during aspirin therapy. Stroke prevention in atrial fibrillation investigators. *Journal of the American College of Cardiology.* 2000;35(1):183–187.

193   Lip GY. Does paroxysmal atrial fibrillation confer a paroxysmal thromboembolic risk? *Lancet.* 1997;349(9065):1565–1566.

194   Petersen P, Godtfredsen J. Embolic complications in paroxysmal atrial fibrillation. *Stroke.* 1986;17(4): 622–626.

195   UK Resuscitation Council. *Advanced Life Support (ALS) Provider Manual* (4th edition) London: Resuscitation Council (UK) Trading Ltd;2004.

196   Strasberg B, Sagie A, Rechavia E et al. Deleterious effects of intravenous verapamil in Wolff–Parkinson–White patients and atrial fibrillation. *Cardiovascular Drugs & Therapy.* 1989;2(6):801–806.

197   Wang HE, O'Connor RE, Megargel RE et al. The use of diltiazem for treating rapid atrial fibrillation in the out-of-hospital setting. *Annals of Emergency Medicine.* 2001;37(1):38–45.

198   Kumar A. Intravenous amiodarone for therapy of atrial fibrillation and flutter in critically ill patients with severely depressed left ventricular function. *Southern Medical Journal.* 1996;89(8):779–785.

199   Faniel R, Schoenfeld P. Efficacy of i.v. amiodarone in converting rapid atrial fibrillation and flutter to sinus rhythm in intensive care patients. *European Heart Journal.* 1983;4(3):180–185.

200   Strasberg B, Arditti A, Sclarovsky S. Efficacy of intravenous amiodarone in the management of paroxysmal or new atrial fibrillation with fast ventricular response. *International Journal of Cardiology.* 1985;7(1):47–55.

201   Stoddard MF, Dawkins PR, Prince CR et al. Left atrial appendage thrombus is not uncommon in patients with acute atrial fibrillation and a recent embolic event: a transesophageal echocardiographic study. *Journal of the American College of Cardiology.* 1995;25(2):452–459.

202 Singer DE, Albers GW, Dalen JE et al. Antithrombotic therapy in atrial fibrillation: the Seventh ACCP Conference on Antithrombotic and Thrombolytic Therapy. *Chest.* 2004;126(3 Suppl):429S–456S.

203 Vecht RJ, Nicolaides EP, Ikweuke JK et al. Incidence and prevention of supraventricular tachy-arrhythmias after coronary bypass surgery. *International Journal of Cardiology.* 1986;13(2):125–134.

204 Creswell LL, Schuessler RB, Rosenbloom M et al. Hazards of postoperative atrial arrhythmias. *Annals of Thoracic Surgery.* 1993;56(3):539–549.

205 Almassi GH, Schowalter T, Nicolosi AC et al. Atrial fibrillation after cardiac surgery: a major morbid event? *Annals of Surgery.* 1997;226(4):501–511.

206 Likosky DS, Caplan LR, Weintraub RM et al. Intraoperative and postoperative variables associated with strokes following cardiac surgery. *Heart Surgery Forum.* 2004;7(4):E271–E276.

207 Maisel WH, Rawn JD, Stevenson WG. Atrial fibrillation after cardiac surgery. *Annals of Internal Medicine.* 2001;135(12):1061–1073.

208 Di Biasi P, Scrofani R, Paje A et al. Intravenous amiodarone vs propafenone for atrial fibrillation and flutter after cardiac operation. *European Journal of Cardio-Thoracic Surgery.* 1995;9(10):587–591.

209 Ryan TJ, Antman EM, Brooks NH. *ACC/AHA guidelines for the management of patients with acute myocardial infarction: a report of the American College of Cardiology/American Heart Association Task Force on Practice Guidelines. Journal of the American College of Cardiology.* 1996;28:1328–1428.

210 Auer J, Weber T, Berent R et al. Serum potassium level and risk of postoperative atrial fibrillation in patients undergoing cardiac surgery. *Journal of the American College of Cardiology.* 2004;44(4):938–939.

211 Miller S, Crystal E, Garfinkle M et al. Effects of magnesium on atrial fibrillation after cardiac surgery: a meta-analysis. *Heart* (British Cardiac Society). 2005;91(5):618–623.

212 Crystal E, Connolly SJ, Ginger T et al. Interventions for preventing postoperative atrial fibrillation in patients undergoing heart surgery. *The Cochrane Library.* 2003;(4)

213 Amar D, Roistacher N, Rusch VW et al. Effects of diltiazem prophylaxis on the incidence and clinical outcome of atrial arrhythmias after thoracic surgery. *Journal of Thoracic & Cardiovascular Surgery.* 2000;120(4):790–798.

214 Van Mieghem W, Tits G, Demuynck K et al. Verapamil as prophylactic treatment for atrial fibrillation after lung operations. *Annals of Thoracic Surgery.* 1996;61(4):1083–1085.

215 Borgeat A, Biollaz J, Bayer-Berger M et al. Prevention of arrhythmias by flecainide after noncardiac thoracic surgery. *Annals of Thoracic Surgery.* 1989;48(2):232–234.

216 Amar D, Roistacher N, Burt ME et al. Effects of diltiazem versus digoxin on dysrhythmias and cardiac function after pneumonectomy. *Annals of Thoracic Surgery.* 1997;63(5):1374–1381.

217 Bayliff CD, Massel DR, Inculet RI et al. Propranolol for the prevention of postoperative arrhythmias in general thoracic surgery. *Annals of Thoracic Surgery.* 1999;67(1):182–186.

218 Lanza LA, Visbal AI, DeValeria PA et al. Low-dose oral amiodarone prophylaxis reduces atrial fibrillation after pulmonary resection. *Annals of Thoracic Surgery.* 2003;75(1):223–230.

219 Reddy P, Dunn AB, White CM et al. An economic analysis of amiodarone versus placebo for the prevention of atrial fibrillation after open heart surgery. *Pharmacotherapy.* 2002;22(1):75–80.

220 Reddy P, Richerson M, Freeman-Bosco L et al. Cost-effectiveness of amiodarone for prophylaxis of atrial fibrillation in coronary artery bypass surgery. *American Journal of Health-System Pharmacy.* 1999;56(21):2211–2217.

221 Mahoney EM, Thompson TD, Veledar E et al. Cost-effectiveness of targeting patients undergoing cardiac surgery for therapy with intravenous amiodarone to prevent atrial fibrillation. *Journal of the American College of Cardiology.* 2002;40(4):737–745.

222 Daoud EG, Strickberger SA, Man KC et al. Preoperative amiodarone as prophylaxis against atrial fibrillation after heart surgery. *New England Journal of Medicine.* 1997;337(25):1785–1791.

223 Stamou SC, Hill PC, Sample GA et al. Prevention of atrial fibrillation after cardiac surgery: the significance of postoperative oral amiodarone. *Chest.* 2001;120(6):1936–1941.

224 Katariya K, DeMarchena E, Bolooki H. Oral amiodarone reduces incidence of postoperative atrial fibrillation. *Annals of Thoracic Surgery.* 1999;68(5):1599–1603.

225 Kim MH, Rachwal W, McHale C et al. Effect of amiodarone +/- diltiazem +/- beta blocker on frequency of atrial fibrillation, length of hospitalization, and hospital costs after coronary artery bypass grafting. *American Journal of Cardiology.* 2002;89(9):1126–1128.

226 Auer J, Weber T, Berent R et al. A comparison between oral antiarrhythmic drugs in the prevention of atrial fibrillation after cardiac surgery: the pilot study of prevention of postoperative atrial fibrillation (SPPAF), a randomized, placebo-controlled trial. *American Heart Journal.* 2004;147(4):636–643.

227 Kalus JS, White CM, Caron MF et al. Indicators of atrial fibrillation risk in cardiac surgery patients on prophylactic amiodarone. *Annals of Thoracic Surgery.* 2004;77(4):1288–1292.

228 Kluger J, White CM. Amiodarone prevents symptomatic atrial fibrillation and reduces the risk of cerebrovascular accidents and ventricular tachycardia after open heart surgery: results of the Atrial Fibrillation Suppression Trial (AFIST). *Cardiac Electrophysiology Review.* 2003;7(2):165–167.

229 Inoue H. Cost-effectiveness of antiarrhythmic drugs for prevention of thromboembolism in patients with paroxysmal atrial fibrillation. *Japanese Circulation Journal.* 2001;65(9):765–768.

230 Tokmakoglu H, Kandemir O, Gunaydin S et al. Amiodarone versus digoxin and metoprolol combination for the prevention of postcoronary bypass atrial fibrillation. *European Journal of Cardio-Thoracic Surgery.* 2002;21(3):401–405.

231 White CM, Giri S, Tsikouris JP et al. A comparison of two individual amiodarone regimens to placebo in open heart surgery patients. *Annals of Thoracic Surgery.* 2002;74(1):69–74.

232 Redle JD, Khurana S, Marzan R et al. Prophylactic oral amiodarone compared with placebo for prevention of atrial fibrillation after coronary artery bypass surgery. *American Heart Journal.* 1999;138(1 Pt 1):144–150.

233 Yazicioglu L, Eryilmaz S, Sirlak M et al. The effect of preoperative digitalis and atenolol combination on postoperative atrial fibrillation incidence. *European Journal of Cardio-Thoracic Surgery.* 2002;22(3): 397–401.

234 Coleman CI, Perkerson KA, Gillespie EL et al. Impact of prophylactic postoperative (beta)-blockade on post-cardiothoracic surgery, length of stay and atrial fibrillation. *Annals of Pharmacotherapy.* 2004; 38(12):2012–2016.

235 Kowey PR, Taylor JE, Rials SJ et al. Meta-analysis of the effectiveness of prophylactic drug therapy in preventing supraventricular arrhythmia early after coronary artery bypass grafting. *American Journal of Cardiology.* 1992;69(9):963–965.

236 Matsuura K, Takahara Y, Sudo Y et al. Effect of sotalol in the prevention of atrial fibrillation following coronary artery bypass grafting. *Japanese Journal of Thoracic & Cardiovascular Surgery.* 2001;49(10): 614–617.

237 Malhotra R, Mishra M, Kler TS et al. Cardioprotective effects of diltiazem infusion in the perioperative period. *European Journal of Cardio-Thoracic Surgery.* 1997;12(3):420–427.

238 Seitelberger R, Hannes W, Gleichauf M et al. Effects of diltiazem on perioperative ischemia, arrhythmias, and myocardial function in patients undergoing elective coronary bypass grafting. *Journal of Thoracic & Cardiovascular Surgery.* 1994;107(3):811–821.

239 Hannes W, Fasol R, Zajonc H et al. Diltiazem provides anti-ischemic and anti-arrhythmic protection in patients undergoing coronary bypass grafting. *European Journal of Cardio Thoracic Surgery.* 1993;7(5): 239–245.

240 Keilich M, Kulinna C, Seitelberger R et al. Postoperative follow-up of coronary artery bypass patients receiving calcium antagonist diltiazem. *International Journal of Angiology.* 1997;6:8–12.

241 Ferraris VA, Ferraris SP, Gilliam H et al. Verapamil prophylaxis for postoperative atrial dysrhythmias: a prospective, randomized, double-blind study using drug level monitoring. *Annals of Thoracic Surgery.* 1987;43(5):530–533.

242 Kowey PR, Yannicelli D, Amsterdam E et al. Effectiveness of oral propafenone for the prevention of atrial fibrillation after coronary artery bypass grafting. *American Journal of Cardiology.* 2004;94(5):663–665.

243 Gold MR, O'Gara PT, Buckley MJ et al. Efficacy and safety of procainamide in preventing arrhythmias after coronary artery bypass surgery. *American Journal of Cardiology.* 1996;78(9):975–979.

244 Laub GW, Janeira L, Muralidharan S et al. Prophylactic procainamide for prevention of atrial fibrillation after coronary artery bypass grafting: a prospective, double-blind, randomized, placebo-controlled pilot study. *Critical Care Medicine.* 1993;21(10):1474–1478.

245 Weiner B, Rheinlander HF, Decker EL et al. Digoxin prophylaxis following coronary artery bypass surgery. *Clinical Pharmacy.* 1986;5(1):55–58.

246 Jakobsen C-J, Bille S, Ahlburg P et al. Perioperative metoprolol reduces the frequency of atrial fibrillation after thoracotomy for lung resection. *Journal of Cardiothoracic & Vascular Anesthesia.* 1997;11(6):746–751.

247 Guo Y, Hu S, Wu Q et al. Predictors of atrial fibrillation after coronary artery bypass graft surgery. *Chinese Medical Journal.* 2002;115(2):232–234.

248 Mathew JP, Fontes ML, Tudor IC et al. A multicenter risk index for atrial fibrillation after cardiac surgery. *Journal of the American Medical Association.* 2004;291(14):1720–1729.

249 Shah P, Shpigel A, Wasser T et al. Morbidity of post-coronary artery bypass surgery patients with atrial fibrillation treated with rate control versus sinus-restoring therapy. *Heartdrug.* 2001;1(4):192–196.

250 Connolly SJ, Mulji AS, Hoffert DL et al. Randomized placebo-controlled trial of propafenone for treatment of atrial tachyarrhythmias after cardiac surgery. *Journal of the American College of Cardiology.* 1987;10(5):1145–1148.

251 Soucier R, Silverman D, Abordo M et al. Propafenone versus ibutilide for postoperative atrial fibrillation following cardiac surgery: neither strategy improves outcomes compared to rate control alone (the PIPAF study). *Medical Science Monitor.* 2003;9(3):I19–I23.

252 Hjelms E. Procainamide conversion of acute atrial fibrillation after open-heart surgery compared with digoxin treatment. *Scandinavian Journal of Thoracic & Cardiovascular Surgery.* 1992;26(3):193–196.

253 Campbell TJ, Gavaghan TP, Morgan JJ. Intravenous sotalol for the treatment of atrial fibrillation and flutter after cardiopulmonary bypass. Comparison with disopyramide and digoxin in a randomised trial. *British Heart Journal.* 1985;54(1):86–90.

254 Cochrane AD, Siddins M, Rosenfeldt FL et al. A comparison of amiodarone and digoxin for treatment of supraventricular arrhythmias after cardiac surgery. *European Journal of Cardio-Thoracic Surgery.* 1994;8(4):194–198.

255 Wafa SS, Ward DE, Parker DJ et al. Efficacy of flecainide acetate for atrial arrhythmias following coronary artery bypass grafting. *American Journal of Cardiology.* 1989;63(15):1058–1064.

256 Lee JK, Klein GJ, Krahn AD et al. Rate control versus conversion strategy in postoperative atrial fibrillation: trial design and pilot study results. *Cardiac Electrophysiology Review.* 2003;7(2):178–184.

257 Williams E, Ansari M, Lip G. Managing atrial fibrillation in the accident and emergency department. *Quarterly Journal of Medicine.* 2001;94(11):609–614.

258 Anon. Secondary prevention in non-rheumatic atrial fibrillation after transient ischaemic attack or minor stroke. *Lancet.* 1993;342(8882):1255–1262.

259 Evans A, Perez I, Yu G et al. Should stroke subtype influence anticoagulation decisions to prevent recurrence in stroke patients with atrial fibrillation? *Stroke.* 2001;32(12):2828–2832.

260 Hart RG, Palacio S, Pearce LA. Atrial fibrillation, stroke, and acute antithrombotic therapy: analysis of randomized clinical trials. *Stroke.* 2002;33(11):2722–2727.

261 Lin H, Wolf PA, Kelly-Hayes M et al. Stroke severity in atrial fibrillation: the Framingham Study. *Stroke.* 1996;27(10):1760–1764.

262 Jorgensen HS, Nakayama H, Reith J et al. Acute stroke with atrial fibrillation: the Copenhagen Stroke Study. *Stroke.* 1996;27(10):1765–1769.

263 Morocutti C, Amabile G, Fattapposta F et al. Indobufen versus warfarin in the secondary prevention of major vascular events in nonrheumatic atrial fibrillation. SIFA (Studio Italiano Fibrillazione Atriale) Investigators 62. *Stroke.* 1997;28(5):1015–1021.

264 Diener HC. Antiplatelet therapy to prevent stroke: risk of brain hemorrhage and efficacy in atrial fibrillation. *Journal of the Neurological Sciences.* 1997;153(1):112.

265 Harenberg J, Weuster B, Pfitzer M et al. Prophylaxis of embolic events in patients with atrial fibrillation using low molecular weight heparin. *Seminars in Thrombosis & Hemostasis.* 1993;19(Suppl 1):116–121.

266 Saxena R. Anticoagulants for preventing stroke in patients with nonrheumatic atrial fibrillation and a history of stroke or transient ischemic attacks. *The Cochrane Library.* 2004;(Issue 4)

267 Hart RG, Pearce LA, Koudstaal PJ. Transient ischemic attacks in patients with atrial fibrillation: implications for secondary prevention: the European Atrial Fibrillation Trial and Stroke Prevention in Atrial Fibrillation III Trial. *Stroke.* 2004;35(4):948–951.

268 DiMarco JP, Flaker GC, Waldo A. Factors affecting bleeding risk during anticoagulant therapy in patients with atrial fibrillation: observations from the Atrial Fibrillation Follow-up Investigation of Rhythm Management (AFFIRM) Study. *American Heart Journal.* 2005;149(4):650–656.

269 Silber S, Albertsson P, Aviles FF et al. Guidelines for percutaneous coronary interventions: the task force for percutaneous coronary interventions of the European Society of Cardiology. *European Heart Journal.* 2005;26(8):804–847.

270 Shireman TI, Howard PA, Kresowik TF et al. Combined anticoagulant–antiplatelet use and major bleeding events in elderly atrial fibrillation patients. *Stroke.* 2004;35(10):2362–2367.

271 Gullov AL, Koefoed BG, Petersen P. Bleeding during warfarin and aspirin therapy in patients with atrial fibrillation: the AFASAK 2 study (Atrial Fibrillation Aspirin and Anticoagulation). *Archives of Internal Medicine.* 1999;159(12):1322–1328.

272 Pengo V, Legnani C, Noventa F et al. Oral anticoagulant therapy in patients with nonrheumatic atrial fibrillation and risk of bleeding. A multicenter inception cohort study. *Thrombosis & Haemostasis.* 2001;85(3):418–422.

273 Anon. Bleeding during antithrombotic therapy in patients with atrial fibrillation. The Stroke Prevention in Atrial Fibrillation Investigators. *Archives of Internal Medicine.* 1996;156(4):409–416.

274 Copland M, Walker ID, Tait RC. Oral anticoagulation and hemorrhagic complications in an elderly population with atrial fibrillation. *Archives of Internal Medicine.* 2001;161(17):2125–2128.

275 Sam C, Massaro JM, D'Agostino RB, Sr. et al. Warfarin and aspirin use and the predictors of major bleeding complications in atrial fibrillation (the Framingham Heart Study). *American Journal of Cardiology.* 2004;94(7):947–951.

276 Abdelhafiz AH, Wheeldon NM. Results of an open-label, prospective study of anticoagulant therapy for atrial fibrillation in an outpatient anticoagulation clinic. *Clinical Therapeutics.* 2004;26(9):1470–1478.

277 Fang MC, Chang Y, Hylek EM et al. Advanced age, anticoagulation intensity, and risk for intracranial hemorrhage among patients taking warfarin for atrial fibrillation. *Annals of Internal Medicine.* 2004;141(10):745–752.

278 Wehinger C, Stollberger C, Langer T et al. Evaluation of risk factors for stroke/embolism and of complications due to anticoagulant therapy in atrial fibrillation. *Stroke.* 2001;32(10):2246–2252.

279 Kalra L, Yu G, Perez I et al. Prospective cohort study to determine if trial efficacy of anticoagulation for stroke prevention in atrial fibrillation translates into clinical effectiveness. *British Medical Journal.* 2000;320(7244):1236–1239.

280 Go AS, Hylek EM, Chang Y et al. Anticoagulation therapy for stroke prevention in atrial fibrillation: how well do randomized trials translate into clinical practice? *Journal of the American Medical Association.* 2003;290(20):2685–2692.

281 Hart RG, Pearce LA, McBride R et al. Factors associated with ischemic stroke during aspirin therapy in atrial fibrillation: analysis of 2012 participants in the SPAF I–III clinical trials. The Stroke Prevention in Atrial Fibrillation (SPAF) Investigators. *Stroke.* 1999;30(6):1223–1229.

282 The SPAF III Writing Committee for the Stroke Prevention in Atrial Fibrillation Investigators. Patients with nonvalvular atrial fibrillation at low risk of stroke during treatment with aspirin: Stroke Prevention in Atrial Fibrillation III Study. The SPAF III Writing Committee for the Stroke Prevention in Atrial Fibrillation Investigators. *Journal of the American Geriatrics Society.* 1998;279(16):1273–1277.

283 Wang TJ, Massaro JM, Levy D et al. A risk score for predicting stroke or death in individuals with new-onset atrial fibrillation in the community: the Framingham Heart Study. *Journal of the American Medical Association.* 2003;290(8):1049–1056.

284 Stollberger C, Chnupa P, Abzieher C et al. Mortality and rate of stroke or embolism in atrial fibrillation during long-term follow-up in the embolism in left atrial thrombi (ELAT) study. *Clinical Cardiology.* 2004;27(1):40–46.

285 van Latum JC, Koudstaal PJ, Venables GS et al. Predictors of major vascular events in patients with a transient ischemic attack or minor ischemic stroke and with nonrheumatic atrial fibrillation. European Atrial Fibrillation Trial (EAFT) Study Group. *Stroke.* 1995;26(5):801–806.

286 Petersen P. Risk factors for thromboembolic complications in chronic atrial fibrillation. The Copenhagen AFASAK study. *Archives of Internal Medicine.* 1990;150(4):819–821.

287 Anon. Predictors of thromboembolism in atrial fibrillation: I. Clinical features of patients at risk. The Stroke Prevention in Atrial Fibrillation Investigators. *Annals of Internal Medicine.* 1992;116(1):1–5.

288 Inoue H, Atarashi H. Risk factors for thromboembolism in patients with paroxysmal atrial fibrillation. *American Journal of Cardiology.* 2000;86(8):852–855.

289 Moulton AW, Singer DE, Haas JS. Risk factors for stroke in patients with nonrheumatic atrial fibrillation: a case-control study. *American Journal of Medicine.* 1991;91(2):156–161.

290 Anon. Risk factors for thromboembolism during aspirin therapy in patients with atrial fibrillation: the Stroke Prevention in Atrial Fibrillation Study. *Journal of Stroke and Cerebrovascular Diseases.* 1995;5(3):147–157.

291 Seidl K, Hauer B, Schwick NG et al. Risk of thromboembolic events in patients with atrial flutter. *American Journal of Cardiology.* 1998;82(5):580–583.

292 Anon. Transesophageal echocardiographic correlates of thromboembolism in high-risk patients with nonvalvular atrial fibrillation. The Stroke Prevention in Atrial Fibrillation Investigators Committee on Echocardiography. *Annals of Internal Medicine.* 1998;128(8):639–647.

293 Chang YJ, Ryu SJ, Lin SK. Carotid artery stenosis in ischemic stroke patients with nonvalvular atrial fibrillation. *Cerebrovascular Diseases.* 2002;13(1):16–20.

294 Lip GY, Lowe GD. ABC of atrial fibrillation. Antithrombotic treatment for atrial fibrillation. *British Medical Journal.* 1996;312(7022):45–49.

295 Fuster V, Ryden LE, Asinger RW et al. ACC/AHA/ESC guidelines for the management of patients with atrial fibrillation: a report of the American College of Cardiology/American Heart Association Task Force on practice guidelines and the European Society of Cardiology Committee for Practice Guidelines and Policy Conferences (Committee to Develop Guidelines for the Management of Patients With Atrial Fibrillation), developed in collaboration with the North American Society of Pacing and Electrophysiology. *Journal of the American College of Cardiology.* 2001;38(4):1266i–1266lxx.

296 Gage BF, Waterman AD, Shannon W et al. Validation of clinical classification schemes for predicting stroke: results from the National Registry of Atrial Fibrillation. *Journal of the American Medical Association.* 2001;285(22):2864–2.

297 Eckman MH, Levine HJ, Salem DN et al. Making decisions about antithrombotic therapy in heart disease: decision analytic and cost-effectiveness issues. *Chest.* 1998;114(5 Suppl):699S–714S.

298 Gage BF, Cardinalli AB, Albers GW et al. Cost effectiveness of warfarin and aspirin for prophylaxis of stroke in patients with nonvalvular atrial fibrillation. *Journal of the American Medical Association.* 1995;274(23):1839–1845.

299 Desbiens NA. Deciding on anticoagulating the oldest old with atrial fibrillation: insights from cost-effectiveness analysis. *Journal of the American Geriatrics Society.* 2002;50(5):863–869.

300 Caro JJ, O'Brien JA, Klittich W et al. The economic impact of warfarin prophylaxis in nonvalvular atrial fibrillation. *Disease Management & Clinical Outcomes.* 1997;1(2):54–60.

301 O'Brien CL, Gage BF. Costs and effectiveness of ximelagatran for stroke prophylaxis in chronic atrial fibrillation. *Journal of the American Medical Association.* 2005;293(6):699–706.

302 Lightowlers S MA. Cost-effectiveness of anticoagulation in nonrheumatic atrial fibrillation in the primary prevention of ischemic stroke. *Stroke.* 1998;29(9):1827–1832.

303 Thomson R, Parkin D, Eccles M et al. Decision analysis and guidelines for anticoagulant therapy to prevent stroke in patients with atrial fibrillation (erratum appears in Lancet 2000 Apr 22;355(9213): 1466). *Lancet.* 2000;355(9208):956–962.

304 Gustafsson C, Asplund K, Britton M et al. Cost effectiveness of primary stroke prevention in atrial fibrillation: Swedish national perspective. *British Medical Journal.* 1992;305(6867):1457–1460.

305 Anon. Risk factors for stroke and efficacy of antithrombotic therapy in atrial fibrillation. Analysis of pooled data from five randomized controlled trials (erratum appears in *Arch Intern Med* 1994 Oct 10;154(19):2254). *Archives of Internal Medicine.* 1994;154(13):1449–1457.

306 Murray ET, Fitzmaurice DA, McCahon D. Point of care testing for INR monitoring: where are we now? *British Journal of Haematology.* 2004;127(4):373–378.

307 Eldor A, Schwartz J. Self-management of oral anticoagulants with a whole blood prothrombin-time monitor in elderly patients with atrial fibrillation. *Pathophysiology of Haemostasis & Thrombosis.* 2002;32(3):99–106.

308 Voller H, Glatz J, Taborski U et al. Self-management of Oral Anticoagulation in Nonvalvular Atrial Fibrillation (SMAAF study). *Zeitschrift für Kardiologie.* 2005;94(3):182–186.

309 Piso B, Jimenz–Boj E, Krinninger B et al. The quality of oral anticoagulation before, during and after a period of patient self–management. *Thrombosis Research.* 2002;106(2):101–104.

310 Cosmi B, Palareti G, Carpanedo M et al. Assessment of patient capability to self-adjust oral anticoagulant dose: a multicenter study on home use of portable prothrombin time monitor (COAGUCHECK). *Haematologica.* 2000;85(8):826–831.

311 Koertke H, Minami K, Bairaktaris A et al. INR self-management following mechanical heart valve replacement. *Journal of Thrombosis & Thrombolysis.* 2000;9 Suppl1:S41–5.

312 Watzke HH, Forberg E, Svolba G et al. A prospective controlled trial comparing weekly self-testing and self-dosing with the standard management of patients on stable oral anticoagulation. *Thrombosis & Haemostasis.* 2000;83(5):661–665.

313 Sawicki PT. A structured teaching and self-management program for patients receiving oral anticoagulation. A randomized controlled trial. *Journal of the American Medical Association.* 1999;281: 145–150.

314 Gadisseur APA, Breukink–Engbers WGM, Van Der Meer FJM et al. Comparison of the quality of oral anticoagulant therapy through patient self-management and management by specialized anticoagulation clinics in the Netherlands: a randomized clinical trial. *Archives of Internal Medicine.* 2003;163(21): 2639–2646.

315 Beyth RJ, Quinn L, Landefeld CS. A multicomponent intervention to prevent major bleeding complications in older patients receiving warfarin: a randomized, controlled trial. *Annals of Internal Medicine.* 2000;133(9):687–695.

316 Sunderji R, Gin K, Shalansky K et al. A randomized trial of patient self-managed versus physician-managed oral anticoagulation. *Canadian Journal of Cardiology.* 2004;20(11):1117–1123.

317 Sidhu P, O'Kane HO. Self-managed anticoagulation: results from a two-year prospective randomized trial with heart valve patients. *Annals of Thoracic Surgery.* 2001;72(5):1523–1527.

318 Cromheecke ME, Levi M, Colly LP et al. Oral anticoagulation self-management and management by a specialist anticoagulation clinic: a randomised crossover comparison. *Lancet.* 2000;356(9224):97–102.

319 Fitzmaurice DA, Murray ET, Gee KM et al. A randomised controlled trial of patient self-management of oral anticoagulation treatment compared with primary care management. *Journal of Clinical Pathology.* 2002;55(11):845–849.

320 Horstkotte D, Piper C, Wiemer M. Optimal frequency of patient monitoring and intensity of oral anticoagulation therapy in valvular heart disease. *Journal of Thrombosis & Thrombolysis.* 1998;5 (Suppl 1):S19–S24.

321 Menendez-Jandula B, Souto JC, Oliver A et al. Comparing self-management of oral anticoagulant therapy with clinic management: a randomized trial. *Annals of Internal Medicine.* 2005;142(1):1–14.

322 Heneghan C, onso-Coello P, Garcia-Alamino JM et al. Self-monitoring of oral anticoagulation: a systematic review and meta-analysis. *Lancet.* 2006;367(9508):404–411.

323 Lafata JE, Martin SA, Kaatz S et al. The cost-effectiveness of different management strategies for patients on chronic warfarin therapy. *Journal of General Internal Medicine.* 2000;15(1):31–37.

324 Niiranen S, Lamminen H, Niemi K et al. A cost study of new media supported near oral anticoagulant treatment follow-up. *International Journal of Medical Informatics.* 2003;70(1):19–29.

325 Fitzmaurice DA, Murray ET, McCahon D et al. Self-management of oral anticoagulation: randomised trial. *British Medical Journal.* 2005;331(7524):1057.

326 Fitzmaurice DA, Machin SJ. Recommendations for patients undertaking self-management of oral anticoagulation. *British Medical Journal.* 2001;323(7319):985–989.

327 Bollmann A, Husser D, Steinert R et al. Echocardiographic and electrocardiographic predictors for atrial fibrillation recurrence following cardioversion. *Journal of Cardiovascular Electrophysiology.* 2003;14(10 Suppl):S162–S165.

328 Dittrich HC, Erickson JS, Schneiderman T et al. Echocardiographic and clinical predictors for outcome of elective cardioversion of atrial fibrillation. *American Journal of Cardiology.* 1989;63(3):193–197.

329 Aytemir K, Aksoyek S, Yildirir A et al. Prediction of atrial fibrillation recurrence after cardioversion by p wave signal-averaged electrocardiography. *International Journal of Cardiology.* 1999;70(1):15–21.

330 Okcun B, Yigit Z, Kucukoglu MS et al. Predictors for maintenance of sinus rhythm after cardioversion in patients with nonvalvular atrial fibrillation. *Echocardiography.* 2002;19(5):351–357.

331 Guo XH, Gallagher MM, Poloniecki J et al. Prognostic significance of serial p wave signal-averaged electrocardiograms following external electrical cardioversion for persistent atrial fibrillation: a prospective study. *Pacing and Clinical Electrophysiology.* 2003;26(1 Part 2):299–304.

332 Berry C, Stewart S, Payne EM et al. Electrical cardioversion for atrial fibrillation: outcomes in 'real-life' clinical practice. *International Journal of Cardiology.* 2001;81(1):29–35.

333 Perez Y, Duval AM, Carville C et al. Is left atrial appendage flow a predictor for outcome of cardioversion of nonvalvular atrial fibrillation? A transthoracic and transesophageal echocardiographic study. *American Heart Journal.* 1997;134(4):745–751.

334 Gentili C, Giordano F, Alois A et al. Efficacy of intravenous propafenone in acute atrial fibrillation complicating open-heart surgery. *American Heart Journal.* 1992;123(5):1225–1228.

335 Galperin J, Elizari MV, Chiale PA et al. Pharmacologic reversion of persistent atrial fibrillation with amiodarone predicts long-term sinus rhythm maintenance. *Journal of Cardiovascular Pharmacology & Therapeutics.* 2003;8(3):179–186.

336 Brugada R, Tapscott T, Czernuszewicz GZ et al. Identification of a genetic locus for familial atrial fibrillation. *New England Journal of Medicine.* 1997;336(13):905–911.

337 Anderson JL, Gilbert EM, Alpert BL et al. Prevention of symptomatic recurrences of paroxysmal atrial fibrillation in patients initially tolerating antiarrhythmic therapy: a multicenter, double-blind, crossover study of flecainide and placebo with transtelephonic monitoring. Flecainide Supraventricular Tachycardia Study Group. *Circulation.* 1989;80(6):1557–1570.

338 Kerr CR, Connolly SJ, Abdollah H et al. Canadian trial of physiological pacing: effects of physiological pacing during long-term follow-up. *Circulation.* 2004;109(3):357–362.

339 Lemery R, Guiraudon G. Catheter and surgical ablation strategies in atrial fibrillation: what have we learned? *Current Opinion in Cardiology.* 2005;20(1):26–30.

340 Cox JL. Surgical treatment of atrial fibrillation: a review. *Europace.* 2004;5 Suppl 1:S20–S29.

341 Leitch JW, Klein G, Yee R et al. Sinus node-atrioventricular node isolation: long-term results with the 'corridor' operation for atrial fibrillation. *Journal of the American College of Cardiology.* 1991;17(4):970–975.

342 Marshall HJ, Harris ZI, Griffith MJ et al. Prospective randomized study of ablation and pacing versus medical therapy for paroxysmal atrial fibrillation: effects of pacing mode and mode-switch algorithm. *Circulation.* 1999;99(12):1587–1592.

343 Wood MA, Brown-Mahoney C, Kay GN et al. Clinical outcomes after ablation and pacing therapy for atrial fibrillation: a meta-analysis. *Circulation.* 2000;101(10):1138–1144.

344 Darpo B, Walfridsson H, Aunes M et al. Incidence of sudden death after radiofrequency ablation of the atrioventricular junction for atrial fibrillation. *American Journal of Cardiology.* 1997;80(9):1174–1177.

345 Twidale N, Manda V, Nave K et al. Predictors of outcome after radiofrequency catheter ablation of the atrioventricular node for atrial fibrillation and congestive heart failure. *American Heart Journal.* 1998;136(4 Pt 1):647–657.

346 Wellens HJ, Lau CP, Luderitz B et al. Atrioverter: an implantable device for the treatment of atrial fibrillation. *Circulation.* 1998;98(16):1651–1656.

347 Krittayaphong R, Raungrattanaamporn O, Bhuripanyo K et al. A randomized clinical trial of the efficacy of radiofrequency catheter ablation and amiodarone in the treatment of symptomatic atrial fibrillation. *Journal of the Medical Association of Thailand.* 2003;86 Suppl 1:8–16.

348 Wazni OM, Marrouche NF, Martin DO et al. Radiofrequency ablation versus antiarrhythmic drugs as first-line treatment of symptomatic atrial fibrillation: a randomized trial. *Journal of the American Medical Association.* 2005;293(21):2634–2640.

349 Verma A, Wazni OM, Marrouche NF et al. Pre-existent left atrial scarring in patients undergoing pulmonary vein antrum isolation: an independent predictor of procedural failure. *Journal of the American College of Cardiology.* 2005;45(2):285–292.

350 Lee SH, Tai CT, Hsieh MH et al. Predictors of early and late recurrence of atrial fibrillation after catheter ablation of paroxysmal atrial fibrillation. *Journal of Interventional Cardiac Electrophysiology.* 2004;10(3):221–226.

351 Purerfellner H, Martinek M, Aichinger J et al. Quality of life restored to normal in patients with atrial fibrillation after pulmonary vein ostial isolation. *American Heart Journal.* 2004;148(2):318–325.

352 Husser D, Bollmann A, Kang S et al. Effectiveness of catheter ablation for coexisting atrial fibrillation and atrial flutter. *American Journal of Cardiology.* 2004;94(5):666–668.

353 Oral H, Knight BP, Tada H et al. Pulmonary vein isolation for paroxysmal and persistent atrial fibrillation. *Circulation.* 2002;105(9):1077–1081.

354 Adragao P, Cavaco D., Reis SK et al. Percutaneous ablation of atrial fibrillation: assessment of outcomes at 1-year follow-up. *Revista Portuguesa de Cardiologia.* 2003;22(11):1301–1308.

355 Chen MS, Marrouche NF, Khaykin Y et al. Pulmonary vein isolation for the treatment of atrial fibrillation in patients with impaired systolic function. *Journal of the American College of Cardiology.* 2004;43(6):1004–1009.

356 Levy T, Walker S, Rochelle J et al. Evaluation of biatrial pacing, right atrial pacing, and no pacing in patients with drug refractory atrial fibrillation. *American Journal of Cardiology.* 1999;84(4):426–429.

357 Fragakis N, Shakespeare CF, Lloyd G et al. Reversion and maintenance of sinus rhythm in patients with permanent atrial fibrillation by internal cardioversion followed by biatrial pacing. *Pacing and Clinical Electrophysiology.* 2002;25(3):278–286.

358 Kawaguchi AT, Kosakai Y, Sasako Y et al. Risks and benefits of combined maze procedure for atrial fibrillation associated with organic heart disease. *Journal of the American College of Cardiology.* 1996;28(4):985–990.

359 Guang Y, Zhen–jie C, Yong LW et al. Evaluation of clinical treatment of atrial fibrillation associated with rheumatic mitral valve disease by radiofrequency ablation. *European Journal of Cardio-Thoracic Surgery.* 2002;21(2):249–254.

360 Handa N, Schaff HV, Morris JJ et al. Outcome of valve repair and the Cox maze procedure for mitral regurgitation and associated atrial fibrillation. *Journal of Thoracic & Cardiovascular Surgery.* 1999;118(4): 628–635.

361 Akpinar B, Guden M, Sagbas E et al. Combined radiofrequency modified maze and mitral valve procedure through a port access approach: early and mid-term results. *European Journal of Cardio-Thoracic Surgery.* 2003;24(2):223–230.

362 Jessurun ER, van Hemel NM, Defauw JJ et al. A randomized study of combining maze surgery for atrial fibrillation with mitral valve surgery. *Journal of Cardiovascular Surgery.* 2003;44(1):9–18.

363 Deneke T, Khargi K, Grewe PH et al. Efficacy of an additional maze procedure using cooled-tip radiofrequency ablation in patients with chronic atrial fibrillation and mitral valve disease. A randomized, prospective trial. *European Heart Journal.* 2002;23(7):558–566.

364 Khargi K, Deneke T, Haardt H et al. Saline-irrigated, cooled-tip radiofrequency ablation is an effective technique to perform the maze procedure. *Annals of Thoracic Surgery.* 2001;72(3):1090–1095.

365 Velimirovic DB, Petrovic P, Djukic P et al. Corridor procedure – surgical option for treatment of chronic atrial fibrillation in patients undergoing mitral valve replacement. *Cardiovascular Surgery.* 1997;5(3):320–327.

366 Isobe N, Taniguchi K, Oshima S et al. Factors predicting success in cryoablation of the pulmonary veins in patients with chronic atrial fibrillation. *Circulation Journal.* 2004;68(11):999–1003.

367 Kawaguchi AT, Kosakai Y, Isobe F et al. Surgical stratification of patients with atrial fibrillation secondary to organic cardiac lesions. *European Journal of Cardio-Thoracic Surgery.* 1996;10(11):983–989.

368 Kamata J, Kawazoe K, Izumoto H et al. Predictors of sinus rhythm restoration after Cox maze procedure concomitant with other cardiac operations. *Annals of Thoracic Surgery.* 1997;64(2):394–398.

369 Choo SJ, Park NH, Lee SK et al. Excellent results for atrial fibrillation surgery in the presence of giant left atrium and mitral valve disease. *European Journal of Cardio-Thoracic Surgery.* 2004;26(2):336–341.

370 Yuda S, Nakatani S, Isobe F et al. Comparative efficacy of the maze procedure for restoration of atrial contraction in patients with and without giant left atrium associated with mitral valve disease. *Journal of the American College of Cardiology.* 1998;31(5):1097–1102.

371 Geidel S, Ostermeyer J, Lass M et al. Surgical treatment of permanent atrial fibrillation during cardiac surgery using monopolar and bipolar radiofrequency ablation. *Indian Pacing & Electrophysiology Journal.* 2003;3(3):93–100.

372 Chen MC, Chang JP, Chang HW. Preoperative atrial size predicts the success of radiofrequency maze procedure for permanent atrial fibrillation in patients undergoing concomitant valvular surgery. *Chest.* 2004;125(6):2129–2134.

373 Brignole M, Gianfranchi L, Menozzi C et al. Assessment of atrioventricular junction ablation and DDDR mode-switching pacemaker versus pharmacological treatment in patients with severely symptomatic paroxysmal atrial fibrillation: a randomized controlled study. *Circulation.* 1997;96:2617–2624.

374 Ueng KC, Tsai TP, Tsai CF et al. Acute and long-term effects of atrioventricular junction ablation and VVIR pacemaker in symptomatic patients with chronic lone atrial fibrillation and normal ventricular response. *Journal of Cardiovascular Electrophysiology.* 2001;12(3):303–309.

375 Brignole M, Menozzi C, Gianfranchi L et al. Assessment of atrioventricular junction ablation and VVIR pacemaker versus pharmacological treatment in patients with heart failure and chronic atrial fibrillation: a randomized, controlled study. *Circulation.* 1998;98(10):953–960.

376 Gianfranchi L, Brignole M, Menozzi C et al. Progression of permanent atrial fibrillation after atrioventricular junction ablation and dual-chamber pacemaker implantation in patients with paroxysmal atrial tachyarrhythmias. *American Journal of Cardiology.* 1998;81(3):351–354.

377 Ricci R, Quesada A, Pignalberi C et al. Dual defibrillator improves quality of life and decreases hospitalizations in patients with drug refractory atrial fibrillation. *Journal of Interventional Cardiac Electrophysiology.* 2004;10(1):85–92.

378 Burns JL, Sears SF, Sotile R et al. Do patients accept implantable atrial defibrillation therapy? Results from the Patient Atrial Shock Survey of Acceptance and Tolerance (PASSAT) Study. *Journal of Cardiovascular Electrophysiology.* 2004;15(3):286–291.

379 Laupacis A, Albers G, Dalen J et al. Antithrombotic therapy in atrial fibrillation. *Chest.* 1998;114 (5 Suppl):579S–589S.

380 OBrien CL, Gage BF. Costs and effectiveness of ximelagatran for stroke prophylaxis in chronic atrial fibrillation. *Journal of the American Medical Association.* 2005;293(6):699–706.